Physical Health and Well-Being in Mental Health Nursing

Clinical Skills for Practice

Physical Health and Well-Being in Mental Health Nursing

Clinical Skills for Practice

Michael Nash

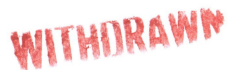
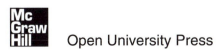

Open University Press

Open University Press
McGraw-Hill Education
McGraw-Hill House
Shoppenhangers Road
Maidenhead
Berkshire
England
SL6 2QL

email: enquiries@openup.co.uk
world wide web: www.openup.co.uk

and Two Penn Plaza, New York, NY 10121-2289, USA

First published 2010

A catalogue record of this book is available from the British Library

ISBN-10: 0 335 23399 6 (pb)   0 335 23398 8 (hb)
ISBN-13: 978 0 335 23399 1 (pb)   978 0 335 23398 4 (hb)

Library of Congress Cataloging-in-Publication Data
CIP data applied for

Typeset by RefineCatch Limited, Bungay, Suffolk
Printed in the UK by Bell and Bain Ltd, Glasgow

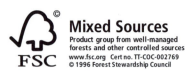

Mixed Sources
Product group from well-managed
forests and other controlled sources
www.fsc.org Cert no. TT-COC-002769
© 1996 Forest Stewardship Council

FSC

The McGraw·Hill Companies

Para mi familia,

mi mujer Maite, y mis hijos Ruben, Érin y Jorge.

Con todo mi amor.

Contents

About the author

Michael Nash is lecturer in psychiatric nursing at Trinity College Dublin. His career began in Gransha Hospital, Derry City before moving to London via a few years in the Channel Islands. In London he worked at various levels in both the NHS and private health care sectors. He studied at the University of North London where he obtained a BSc (Hons) in Health Studies then at St George's Medical School, University of London where he eventually obtained an MSc in Health Sciences. He moved into higher education spending happy years at London Metropolitan University where he obtained a Post-graduate Certificate in Learning and Teaching before moving to Middlesex University. At Middlesex he commenced a professional doctorate that is nearing completion and has retained many good friendships from very happy times there.

Acknowledgements

I would like to thank some colleagues and friends who have helped me through the process of writing this book. First to Nicky Torrance, Jeff Sapiro and Sheila Fawell at Middlesex University, London who gave me the time and space necessary to develop the ideas for the book. To Janet Holmshaw, also at Middlesex, for her support and encouragement during the long process of writing; it was much appreciated. I would also like to thank Professor Agnes Higgins at Trinity College Dublin for her support and understanding when finishing the book.

I would also like to thank those who gave me permission to reproduce their valued work in this book.

Finally, thanks to Rachel for her kind comments and support throughout the lengthy writing and editing process, we got there – eventually.

Abbreviations and acronyms

ABGS	arterial blood gases
ADR	adverse drug reaction
BHF	British Heart Foundation
BLS	basic life support
BMI	body mass index
BNF	British National Formulary
BP	blood pressure
CA	cardiac arrest
CCU	coronary care unit
CHD	coronary heart disease
CMHN	community mental health nurse
COPD	chronic obstructive pulmonary disease
CPA	care programme approach
CNS	central nervous system
DH	Department of Health
DKA	diabetic ketoacidosis
DRC	Disability Rights Commission
DSM IV	Diagnostic and Statistical Manual IV
ECG	electrocardiogram
ECT	electro-convulsive therapy
FBC	full blood count
HDLs	high density lipoproteins
HE	health education
HNA	health needs assessment
HP	health promotion
HPA	Health Protection Agency
ICD 10	International Classification of Diseases 10
IoH	Inequalities of Health
IR	incidence rate
LDLs	low density lipoproteins
LE	life expectancy
MAOIs	monoamine oxidase inhibitors
MHN	mental health nurse
MR	mortality rate
NICE	National Institute of Health and Clinical Excellence
NMC	Nursing and Midwifery Council
NMS	neuroleptic malignant syndrome
NRT	nicotine replacement therapy
NSF	National Service Framework
OH	orthostatic hypotension
OPDM	Office of the Deputy Prime Minister
OT	occupational therapist

PEFR   peak expiratory flow rate
PR   prevalence rate
RT   rapid tranquilisation
SMART   specific, measurable, attainable, realistic and timely
SMI   severe mental illness
SMR   standardized mortality ratio
SS   serotonin syndrome
SSRIs   selective serotonin reuptake inhibitors
STD   sexually transmitted disease
T2D   type 2 diabetes
TNA   training needs analysis
WCC   white cell count
WHO   World Health Organization

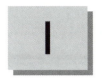

An introduction to physical health in mental illness

By the end of this chapter you should be able to:

- Define health and health beliefs and illustrate why these are important to clients
- Appreciate the impact of physical illness on our clients
- Identify factors that negatively impact on the physical health of our clients
- Be aware of barriers to physical care of our clients

Box 1.1
Exercise

Describe the physical health status of your client group. List the most common physical health problems you encounter.

Physical well-being is important to all of us whether we have a mental health problem or not. Indeed the physical health needs of our clients mirror those of the general population. Physical health of clients has become more prominent in mental health policy and practice arenas. After seemingly years of neglect it became apparent that the physical health of clients under the care of mental health services was not only poor but a largely unaddressed area of need. Nash (2005) suggests that this lack of focus on physical health compromises the notion of holistic care in mental health practice. Therefore physical health must be embraced as part of a holistic assessment that includes social, emotional, economic and psychological needs.

What do we know about physical health in people with severe mental illness?

The focus of this book is the specific issues related to people with a primary mental health problem and a secondary physical problem, e.g. schizophrenia and diabetes. However, we should remain aware that there are issues relating to individuals with a primary physical condition and a secondary mental health problem. The World Health Organization (WHO 2003) suggests high prevalence of co-morbid depression in a range of physical illnesses, for example, depression in hypertension is up to 29 per cent, in cancer up to 33 per cent, in HIV/AIDS up to 44 per cent and in TB up to 46 per cent. This is something community practitioners should be aware of in respect to mental health promotion (MHP) in primary care.

Poor physical health affects our mental well-being while mental illness increases mortality and morbidity. A combination of both can impair the rate or fullness of recovery. Research has consistently shown that the physical health of people with severe mental illness is frequently poor (Phelan *et al.* 2001). This is evidenced by the following:

- There are higher Standardized Mortality Ratios (SMRs) for cardiovascular disease, deaths due to infections and deaths from respiratory disorders (Harris and Barraclough 1998).
- There exists a higher risk of preventable death, with Farnam *et al.* (1999) estimating that people with mental illness die between 10 and 15 years earlier than the general population.
- People with bipolar disorder and diabetes have a 50 per cent higher risk of dying than someone with diabetes who does not have a mental illness (DRC 2006).
- People with schizophrenia may be at increased risk for Type 2 diabetes because of the side effects of medication, poorer healthcare, poor physical health and less healthy lifestyles (Dixon *et al.* 2000).
- In the UK 62 per cent of people with a psychotic disorder reported themselves as having a long-standing physical complaint as compared to 42 per cent with no psychotic disorder (Singleton *et al.* 2000).

The irony is that in many instances these statistics refer to current service users, in contact with either teams of health and social care professionals, or primary care services. We must therefore ask ourselves how can such severe and chronic physical illness be so prevalent in our client group and yet go undetected? This is not just a question for specialist mental health services. It is also a question for primary care services where, in the UK, people with mental health problems have 13 to 14 consultations with their GP per year (Mentality and NIMHE 2004) yet severe and chronic physical conditions are underdiagnosed.

Concerns regarding poor physical health in mental health are not confined to the UK, it is an international problem. For example, in Western Australia Lawrence *et al.* (2001) found that clients died between 1.3 and 5.4 times more than the general population, for all major natural causes of death while in the USA Parks *et al.* (2006) found clients die on average 25 years earlier than the general population.

What is health?

> **Box 1.2 Exercise** How would you define (a) health and (b) illness? Which models might influence your definitions e.g. medical, social or psychological?

It is over fifty years since the World Health Organization (WHO) was established and the most often cited definition of health originates from them. The WHO (1948) defines health as 'a state of complete physical, mental and social well being and not merely the absence of disease or infirmity'. Saracci (1997) suggests that this is more a definition of happiness than health. He cites an anecdote from Sigmund Freud who, on having to stop smoking for health reasons, wrote 'I am now better than I was, but not happier.'

The WHO definition is certainly one to aspire to but it does not appear entirely holistic. It is a twentieth century definition in a twenty-first century world and omits other factors that are now deemed important for positive health, for example, emotional, environmental and spiritual factors – however, the 'social' aspect might encompass these. In developing the National Aboriginal Mental Health Policy and Plan, Swan and Raphael (1995) found that Aboriginal concepts of mental health are holistic being defined as: 'health does not just mean the physical well-being of the individual but refers to the social, emotional and cultural well-being of the whole community'.

Defining health is problematic as individual experiences of health and illness will rarely be the same. Health, and indeed, illness are inherently individualized concepts. For example, have you ever gone to work sick? Why? Maybe you felt that you could struggle on, maybe you didn't want the hassle of reporting sick. Nevertheless through a process of rationalization we may underestimate our levels of illness by saying 'it's only a cold' in order to undertake our other social roles. Similarly we may diminish our own ill health, or have our ill health diminished by others through comparison to other people, e.g. 'at least it's not cancer'.

Another way to explore the question 'what is health?' may be to look at what can make us unhealthy or ill. However, again this is controversial as being labelled unhealthy or ill can be stigmatizing and disempowering. Despite being problematic, defining health is important for developing public health strategy, models of health care delivery and diagnosing illness. Being complex to define, we might suggest that holistic definitions of health based on multidimensional models would be best for exploring both risk factors and protective factors for physical illness.

Blaxter (1990) explored the concept of health by surveying 9000 individuals and asking the following questions: (i) Think of someone you know who is very healthy; who are you thinking of? How old are they and what makes you call them healthy? (ii) At times people are healthier than at other times. What is it like when you are healthy? Ten categories of health and the characteristics that typified the responses are outlined in Table 1.1.

Health beliefs

There will always be a tension between what professionals and the public believe about concepts of health and illness. The health beliefs of the general public will influence their help-seeking behaviour and the health beliefs of professionals influence the types of interventions and services they provide. Indeed health beliefs may vary between cultures, for example, the mind–body split that occurs in Western medicine.

One aspect of mental health that can complicate our understanding of clients' health beliefs is the concept of insight. Insight is a frequently used descriptor in mental health. There is no uniform definition of insight as it is not a black and white issue and commonly used descriptors

Table 1.1 Ten categories of health and the characteristics that typified the responses

Health category	Characteristic
1 Negative answers	Health not rated highly as a virtue, a lack of concern for healthy behaviour
2 Health as not ill	Being symptom free, never seeing a doctor
3 Health as absence of disease/ health despite disease	Did not have any really serious illness, 'I am healthy although I do have diabetes'
4 Health as a reserve	The ability to recover quickly
5 Health as behaviour, as the healthy life	Health defined as 'virtuous' behaviour – being a non-smoker or non-drinker
6 Health as physical fitness	Being athletic or sporty, also for women having a good outward appearance
7 Health as energy, vitality	Having 'get up and go'
8 Health as a social relationship	Health defined as having good relationships with others – especially for women
9 Health as a function	Being able to do things with less stress
10 Health as psychosocial well-being	Health as a state of mind

include: lacks insight; partial insight; insightless or; has insight. These measures are rather vague and do little to enhance our understanding or knowledge of insight. This may limit its therapeutic value. We may not know what insight is, but we know when it is not there. Although frequently used in relation to schizophrenia, insight is not a diagnostic category for schizophrenia in the International Classification of Disease 10 (ICD 10).

Having insight means that a person is aware that they are ill, that they need to get help and accept treatment. Gelder *et al.* (1996: 23) define insight as 'awareness of ones own medical condition'. When someone does not have insight they do not recognize they are ill or that they need treatment. Amador (2001) approaches insight in neurological terms – anosognosia – meaning 'unawareness of illness', while David (1990) proposes that insight is composed of three distinct, overlapping dimensions, namely, the recognition that one has a mental illness, compliance with treatment, and the ability to re-label, or attribute, unusual mental events (e.g. delusions and hallucinations) as pathological.

Box 1.3 Case example

Farlo has a 20 year history of schizophrenia. He presents with two main psychotic symptoms – auditory hallucinations and delusions of grandeur. He refuses to accept treatment, maintaining he is not sick. This is confirmed by TV news reports which say he is doing well. 'How can I the great, supreme and magical Farlo be unwell?' he asks the team at the ward round. Farlo currently lacks insight as (a) he is unaware that he is unwell; (b) he does not see the need for treatment; and (c) he does not attribute his psychotic symptoms to a mental illness.

Health beliefs, on the other hand, are our individually held beliefs about our own health and illness status – what causes us to be healthy, what may cause us to be ill, what we must do to stay well or what we must do in order to recover. While these are individual they have also been found to be social as they can be influenced by social factors such as culture (Herzlich 1973). A recurring problem with health beliefs is that clients may not share these with health providers or, in the case of smoking, they share the view that smoking is dangerous but continue to smoke. This clash of beliefs can be very challenging to the development and maintenance of therapeutic relationships, especially in mental health care with the added complexity of insight.

Linden and Godemann (2005) in a study of 364 schizophrenic outpatients assessed lack of insight and health beliefs and found these to be independent of each other. This meant that insight was related to their illness and health beliefs were related to personal life experiences. Although both concepts are associated with patient non-compliance, Linden and Godemann state that they are 'separate clinical phenomena' and as such this distinction should be made. This means that practitioners should not attribute poor lifestyle choices to a lack of insight. It is important for practitioners to know and understand the health beliefs of clients in order to better implement health education (HE) and health promotion interventions. It is also important not to conflate health beliefs with insight as health beliefs will influence responses to health and also the therapeutic nurse-patient relationship.

Box 1.4 Case example

Ruari has a ten year history of schizo-affective disorder. He is currently in hospital due to a relapse caused by non-compliance with antipsychotic medications. Ruari also has a history of asthma and uses a bronchodilator. At medication rounds he willingly accepts his asthma medication but staff need to continually prompt and encourage him to take his antipsychotic medication. When he is asked why he takes one medication and not the other Ruari replies 'I have asthma and need my puffer to help me breathe. I even cut down on my smoking. But everyone tells me I'm mentally ill and I need to take the other tablets, but I don't feel sick. Mentally I feel fine.'

Ruari is unaware that he has a mental illness as he appears to lack insight. Yet Ruari's health beliefs indicate that he is aware of the need to take asthma medication and that he has even reduced his smoking. His health beliefs seem to be in conflict with insight. However, we must not conflate these as they are separate factors in health and illness. What practitioners need to do is use Ruari's health beliefs about his asthma as a metaphor for his mental illness – the need to take treatment and keep taking it. Ruari may then accept that he requires antipsychotic medication to keep him well, just as he requires his bronchodilator for his asthma.

Physical illness will seldom be caused by one factor, rather it will be an interaction of many risk factors. The challenge for practitioners is to have the knowledge of the risk factors and skills to assess – either for screening or further investigation – using appropriate clinical skills and techniques. However, a further challenge for us is being able to implement the same process across a range of physical conditions prevalent in our clients, e.g. obesity or diabetes.

Factors that influence physical health in people with mental illness

The UK government states the reality of health inequality very clearly when it says 'the poorer you are, the more likely you are to be ill and to die younger' (DH 1999a). This is truer for our clients in a range of physical conditions. However, the government still places some emphasis on the individual's responsibility for improving their own health through physical activity, an improved diet and quitting smoking (DH 1999a). Therefore, while health beliefs play an important role in our decision making, there are three important influences on the physical health of clients:

- Lifestyle factors
- Social factors
- Adverse drug reactions

The impact of lifestyle factors on the physical health of clients

The lifestyle choices we make can directly impact, positively or negatively, on our health. If someone smokes they face an increased risk of ill health or if they exercise and eat healthily they reduce the risk of ill health. Our clients are often exposed to adverse lifestyle choices for example:

- Smoking prevalence is significantly higher among people with mental health problems than the general population. Some studies show rates as high as 80 per cent among people with schizophrenia (McNeill 2001).
- Kendrick (1996) found that of 101 people with SMI living in the community 26 were clinically obese.
- McCreadie et al. (1998) found that people with schizophrenia made poor dietary choices characterized by a high fat, low fibre dietary intake.

- Lifestyle factors that cause obesity, such as low levels of exercise and poor diet, are present in people with mental illness (Brown *et al.* 1999).

The outcomes of unhealthy lifestyle choices are increased risk of developing severe and chronic long term physical conditions such as type two diabetes, coronary heart disease (CHD), stroke or smoking related respiratory disorders. However, people need to be fully informed about the risks of making unhealthy decisions and research shows that clients seldom receive the same health promotion advice or interventions as the general population (Burns and Cohen 1998). The result is a double whammy of an SMI and a chronic physical problem which can serve to exclude clients from employment or educational opportunities where they may be too ill to avail themselves of these.

How can social factors influence the physical health of our clients?

Having a diagnosis of mental illness negatively impacts on the client's socio-economic circumstances. A UK government report *The Social and Economic Circumstances of Adults with Mental Disorders* (Meltzer *et al.* 2002) found the following:

- Compared with all other groups, those with a psychotic disorder were more likely to have left school before reaching 16 years of age, without qualifications.
- About 60 per cent of the sample assessed as having a psychotic disorder lived in a household with an income less than £300 a week compared with 37 per cent of those with a current neurotic disorder and 28 per cent with no mental disorder.
- Those with a mental disorder were far more likely than those with no disorder to be living in rented accommodation (38 per cent compared with 24 per cent).
- Three of these six specified life events were twice as likely to have been experienced by those with a mental disorder compared with those with no mental disorder: separation or divorce (44 per cent compared with 23 per cent); serious injury, illness or assault (40 per cent compared with 22 per cent); and having a serious problem with a close friend or relative (27 per cent compared with 13 per cent).

Box 1.5   What factors do you consider are important in determining our health status?
Exercise

Determinants of health

Wanless (2004) suggests that health and well-being are influenced by many factors including past and present behaviour, healthcare provision and 'wider determinants' including social, cultural and environmental factors. While it is accepted that lifestyle factors are important in determining physical health, practitioners should not overlook other important factors such as social class.

People living in the poorest part of society will be more exposed to determinants of ill health, especially those living in inner city areas where there is an increased exposure to poverty, social deprivation and social exclusion. Typically these neighbourhoods have poor housing, few leisure amenities, higher levels of unemployment and increased crime or the threat of crime and reduced access to education and low educational attainment, for example, more school expulsions.

The UK government recognizes that health inequality is widespread and the most disadvantaged have suffered most from poor health (DH 1999a). Therefore while this type of environment is not conducive to good health, it is the type of environment where many of our clients will come from. This should prompt us to be more aware of the influence of social factors on physical health.

Inequalities in health

While lifestyle factors offer a biological explanation of health and illness, the social model can offer us alternative explanations. One important factor in the health of any population is Inequalities of Health (IoH). Acheson (1998) contends that where IoH exist we can see great differences in health status in social classes when using occupation as a measurement. This is illustrated by health gradients where those in lower social classes tend to have poorer health (increased morbidity) and poorer health outcomes (increased mortality). The UK Department of Health (2008a) states that health inequalities are the result of a complex and wide-ranging network of factors such as material disadvantage, poor housing, lower educational attainment, insecure employment or homelessness. People exposed to IoH have poorer health outcomes and an earlier death compared with the rest of the population.

Our clients are a socially disenfranchised group, often excluded from the fundamental aspects of society (Nash 2002). Therefore an alternative explanation for a client's poor physical health is their position in the social hierarchy. Coming from the lowest social class they face greater morbidity and mortality than those from higher social classes. This offers us an alternative explanation to lifestyle factors. Figures 1.1 and 1.2 illustrate the class gradient in respect to death rates in general (Figure 1.1) and deaths by suicide (Figure 1.2).

Social class and mental illness

People with mental health problems are often over represented in the lower social classes. Those with psychotic disorders are more likely to be of a lower social class (see Table 1.2). The Public Health Agency of Canada (2002) nicely illustrates two theories for this:

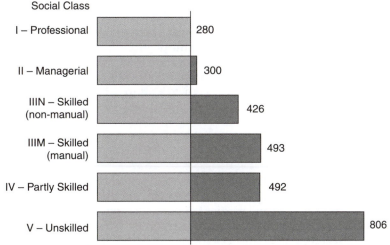

European standardized mortality rate per 100,000 population
for men aged 20–64 in England and Wales, 1991–93

Figure 1.1 Social class and mortality

Source: (DH 1999a)

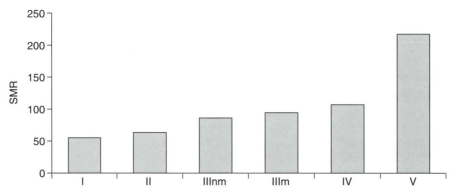

Figure 1.2 Social class and suicide: men aged 20–64, England 1997
Source: DH (2002a)

Table 1.2 Social class and mental illness

	Psychotic disorder	**No psychotic disorder**
Social Class IV or V	39%	22%
Economically Inactive	70%	30%

Source: Office of National Statistics (2000)

- 'Social drift': this theory suggests that individuals who are predisposed to mental illness have lower than expected educational and occupational attainment and therefore 'drift' down the socio-economic ladder.
- 'Social causation': this theory suggests that social experiences of members of different socio-economic groups influence the likelihood of becoming mentally ill, e.g. members of lower social classes are subjected to greater stress as a result of deprivation and are forced to cope with elevated stress levels with limited resources.

Social class can affect the prevalence of mental health problems. Here we can see the part that poverty and deprivation has in influencing the physical and mental health of socially excluded groups. Therefore the challenge to practitioners is clear. The majority of our client group will come from a backdrop of adverse social conditions with experiences of poverty and deprivation. We should therefore be aware that there is a strong likelihood that our clients from this group will have a physical health condition that may be undiagnosed or may be at risk of developing one.

Poverty

Mental illness seldom discriminates between class, gender or ethnicity and the WHO (2003: 7) states that no group is immune to mental disorders, but the risk is higher among the poor, the homeless, the unemployed and persons with low education. Poverty is an important factor in physical and mental ill health. In Ireland a report by Walsh and Daly (2004) suggested that social class divisions indicate that poverty and disadvantage are contributory factors, both to the incidence and prevalence of mental illness. In the UK a survey by Focus on Mental Health (2001) found that clients suffered significant poverty as a result of not being able to get work. It also asked clients about their experiences of living on a low income and found the following:

- 66 per cent of respondents had difficulties making their income last for a week.
- 81 per cent of respondents thought that mental health problems increased the likelihood of being on low income.
- 50 per cent of respondents said that their financial situation meant they were excluded from their community.

Employment

Employment is seen as a way out of poverty. Being in work increases our quality of life through material wealth and economic productivity. Employment can also increase our self-worth and self-esteem and it can protect us against social exclusion. Employment is a key priority for clients and a key component of recovery. However, research shows that only around 20 per cent of people with mental health problems are in employment (DRC 2006), while the Social Exclusion Unit (2004) found that mental health problems are more likely to be listed on GP sickness certificates in the most deprived areas of the country.

Clients frequently encounter discrimination and negative, stereotypical attitudes among employers. Research by the DRC (2003) found that only around 37 per cent of employers are willing to take on someone with a mental health problem while the Social Exclusion Unit found clients experience stigma as a barrier to employment (ODPM 2004).

Lacking employment opportunities means that our clients depend on social welfare benefits. This places them in the lowest income group, which the UK government recognizes is clearly linked to ill health (DH 1999a). Therefore, while clients battle established stigma and discrimination, they may be doing so in a state of poor physical health. This may constitute another barrier to gainful employment as clients want to work but are physically unable to. These social factors tend to snowball and trap clients in a vicious cycle of poverty and deprivation. This increases their risk of social exclusion and poor health outcomes.

Social inclusion and social exclusion

The preceding parts of this chapter serve to build up a picture of how social factors can influence the health of clients and their inclusion or exclusion. Social inclusion is defined as 'a virtuous circle of improved rights of access to the social and economic world, new opportunities, recovery of status and meaning and reduced impact of disability' (Sayce 2001: 122). To be included in society means to be accepted as 'one of us', enabling easier access to healthcare services or employment. However, all too often clients are seen as 'one of them' – as outside of society – and face social exclusion. Sayce (2000) defines social exclusion as 'the interlocking and mutually compounding problems of impairment, discrimination, diminished social role, lack of economic and social participation and disability'. Social exclusion often results in decreased social networks, including healthcare networks, which can further exacerbate both mental and physical health problems.

Adverse drug reactions

While this will be covered in detail in Chapter 8, it is worth briefly mentioning this issue here. Iatrogenic illness, illness caused by adverse drug reactions, contributes to physical ill health in our clients. Anti-psychotic medication has side effects that can lead to obesity, increased risk of developing type 2 diabetes and cardiac problems. This is quite different from lifestyle or social factors as it is a risk factor unique to our clients. Members of the general population will not be exposed to this risk factor.

So far we have examined factors that influence the physical health of our clients. These factors will seldom be stand alone and most probably will be interlinked. Poor lifestyle can naturally increase the risk of ill health but lifestyle choices may be restricted by social factors such as social class, inequalities in health and social exclusion. Adverse drug reactions also increase the risk of physical illness for clients. However, there is a final piece of the puzzle of factors that can increase physical illness in clients and we will now explore this.

Box 1.6 **Exercise**	Revisit your answer to exercise three above. Which other factors can act as barriers to physical health care in your client group?

Barriers to physical health care for clients

By far one of the most problematic areas of mental health care is stigma. In the 2007 Attitudes to Mental Illness survey for the UK Department of Health (TNS 2007) there was an overall decrease in positive attitudes towards people with mental illness since 1994. This may be due to the frequency of reports into incidents involving people with mental illness in the community during this period and how these were reported in the media.

However, having negative attitudes about people with mental illness is not confined to the general public. Research shows that health professionals, including those in mental health care, can harbour stereotypical or stigmatizing views towards clients. For example in a survey of clients by Mind (1996) one third felt that their GP had treated them unfairly due to their mental illness. With respect to mental health professionals Lewis and Appleby (1988) found that psychiatrists had negative attitudes towards personality disorder finding this client group less deserving of care, manipulative, attention seeking and annoying. In a study of 65 qualified mental health nurses (MHNs) working in both inpatient and community services, Deans and Meocevic (2006) observed that the majority of them found people with borderline personality disorder manipulative with some having negative attitudes towards this client group.

Stigma often prevents people from seeking help to the extent that, when they do, their condition may have significantly worsened. This view is supported by Ward (1997) who found that negative media reporting can negatively impact on an individual's help-seeking behaviour. Yamey (1999) reports the case of a psychiatrist, who during the course of a ward round found that two thirds (four out of six) patients had been struck off their GP's list since admission. Following a further audit of 50 patients it was found that 30 per cent had been removed from their GP's list at some point. This prompted a suspicion that some behavioural and psychiatric disorders could be construed as a reason for being excluded from GP lists.

Healthcare professionals' attitudes

There are some myths and stereotypes surrounding physical health in clients which need to be dispelled in order for progress to be made. We can rightly speculate that having negative and stereotypical views of clients will have an impact in the way that care is provided to, or for, them. This is especially true of physical health care where at times practitioners may have a therapeutic fatalism, for example, 'it's no good trying to get them to stop smoking, they have been doing it for years'. Research by Dean *et al.* (2001) and Meddings and Perkins (2002) shows a prevailing assumption among mental health practitioners that clients are not interested in their physical health when, in fact, they are. This was typified with responses such as 'people have more to worry about (in relation to smoking cessation)'.

Elsewhere it has been reported that some clients report 'inappropriate stereotyping, negative attitudes and detrimental assumptions about the quality of life of people with mental illness' (Nocon and Sayce 2006: 109), while the DRC (2006) found that individual experiences of primary care included reception staff with 'bad' attitudes, clients feeling that their physical symptoms were attributed to their mental illness and a perception of a lack of attention to problems.

Diagnostic overshadowing

As far back as 1979 Koranyi found that major medical illnesses went undiagnosed with clients' physical complaints being labelled as 'psychosomatic'. This process is known as diagnostic overshadowing (DO). DO is essentially a judgement bias, where a physical complaint or symptoms are put down to the mental illness rather than a genuine physical illness.

Box 1.7 Case example

Brian is a 38-year-old male with a 20-year history of paranoid schizophrenia. He has periods of non-compliance with medication and is currently on olanzapine 20 mg BD. He frequently drinks alcohol, but not illicit substances and smokes up to 40 cigarettes daily. He does not exercise and recognizes that his diet is very poor. Brian tells his nurse that he has abdominal pains, saying 'I feel something is growing inside my stomach'. His nurse puts this down to a nihilistic delusion and encourages Brian to continue taking his anti-psychotic medications.

This sounds entirely plausible and the nurse has acted on the presenting clinical picture. However, the likelihood of a physical complaint has been overlooked due to the history of mental illness (DO). Of course people with schizophrenia can have delusions like this but recent evidence from the DRC (2006) shows that people with schizophrenia are 90 per cent more likely – i.e. nearly twice as likely – to get bowel cancer, which is the second most common cause of cancer death in Britain. Therefore what is considered a delusion here may well be a severe physical complaint that needs investigation. We cannot second guess that the investigations might reinforce the delusion without first ruling out a primary physical cause. Delays like this may place Brian at risk of more serious illness, which when finally diagnosed might require radical surgery. If it turns out to be a delusion then we can begin interventions designed to reduce the impact of this.

Lack of policy guidance on responsibilities for clients' physical health

This is not, strictly speaking, true. The UK National Service Framework Mental Health (DH 1999b) advocates the monitoring of physical health of clients both in mental health and primary care services. There are also physical monitoring guidelines attached to the National Institute of Health and Clinical Excellence (NICE) guidelines for bipolar disorder (NICE 2006) and schizophrenia (NICE 2009) respectively. However, there are other National Service Frameworks, for example, coronary heart disease (DH 2000a) or diabetes (DH 2001b) which have population health targets to be reached. How well these have been used as resources and integrated into our mental health practice is highly questionable.

Mental health professionals' skills

Another barrier to physical health for clients is professionals' skills. In a training needs analysis of inpatient and community mental health nurses' physical care skills Nash (2005) found that many of the sample did not have up to date physical care skills or knowledge. This may lead to a lack of confidence at taking on physical care activities or a lack of knowledge of symptoms of physical illness which might delay appropriate intervention. However, other past surveys reported that most psychiatrists did not examine their patients routinely and did not feel competent performing a physical examination (McIntyre and Romano 1977).

Box 1.8   SWOT Analysis
Exercise
Think about your service/clinical area. What are the Strengths, Weaknesses, Opportunities and Threats regarding the physical health of clients? For example, a strength might be a routine physical assessment schedule; a weakness might be the ad hoc implementation of the physical assessment schedule

Conclusion

Being physically well is a goal for many people as good physical health can have a positive impact on psychological health. It is important that the physical health needs of clients are identified and effectively managed. Irrespective of the compulsion in the duty of care to clients, we should have a more vested interest in securing their good physical health. We cannot allow the glaring differences in morbidity and mortality between those with and without mental illness to continue.

Clients, like everyone, are concerned about their physical health, even though at times their lifestyle choices are at variance with this. This serves to illustrate the complex nature of beliefs and behaviours about physical health and illness. We should be hesitant in linking all lifestyle choices to the consequences of having a mental health problem and seek to address the physical health of clients in a truly holistic way. This will mean that we should assume less defeatist attitudes about clients not being able to change nor adopt a 'you can't teach old dogs new tricks' philosophy.

If we really are in the business of holistic care we should be ensuring that physical health issues are addressed as part of the whole system approach to mental health care. This may require innovative practice and the use of what we already know in different ways. We can ensure physical health is integrated into local mental health documentation, e.g. the Care Programme Approach (CPA) in the UK, or advocating more loudly for our clients to have their physical health addressed in primary care settings.

This chapter should make us critically examine the notion that poor health in clients is solely lifestyle factor related. Undoubtedly lifestyle does play a part but all practitioners should continually reflect on their attitudes, approaches to physical care for clients, knowledge and skills and ensure that they have fair and equitable access to physical healthcare services.

Summary of key points

- Clients have poorer physical health and health outcomes than the general population due to inequalities of health and/or poor lifestyle choices.
- Clients are at greater risk of social exclusion which can negatively impact on health status.
- Mental health nurses need to develop a better understanding of clients' health beliefs.
- Attitudes of healthcare professionals towards the physical health of clients may present as a barrier to care.

• Clients are concerned about their physical health status and practitioners should advocate for better physical healthcare services.

Quick quiz

1 Define social exclusion. What effect will social inclusion have on the health status of clients?
2 Describe the types of health inequalities that people with severe mental illness may face. How might these inequalities impact on physical health status?
3 How might the negative attitudes of health care professionals affect the physical care of people with severe mental illness?
4 What barriers to good physical health do clients face?
5 What type of barriers to physical care can you identify for your client group?

2 An introduction to key concepts in measuring health and illness

By the end of this chapter you will be able to:

- Define key terms in health measurement, e.g. incidence, prevalence, standardized mortality ratio and mortality rate

- Illustrate how knowledge of epidemiology can help mental health nurses in practice

- Define demographics

- Discuss risk factors in respect to public health

- Describe the process for screening and profiling caseloads for physical illness

Introduction

Box 2.1 | List the factors that can increase your client's risk of physical illness.
Exercise

In Chapter 1 we discussed the effect of lifestyle factors, social class, health inequalities and adverse drug reactions on clients' physical health. We should be mindful of these factors when profiling our population health as the WHO (2004a) suggest the clearest evidence is associated with indicators of poverty. This includes low levels of education, and in some studies, poor housing and poor income. Increasing and persisting socio-economic disadvantages for individuals and for communities are recognized risks to mental health.

This chapter will explore the epidemiology of physical illness in clients and will probably confirm what you already know from your clinical practice. However, it will strive to put this in the context of available evidence. We will explore the concept of risk, but in a different way from what is typical in mental health. We will consider risk factors for physical illness and how these can be examined and managed through the concept of health needs assessment.

Most of us will have considered the impact of client physical illness on our work. For example, how often do you now provide physical care compared to three years ago? What is the prevalence of diabetes in your client group or the incidence of problems associated with smoking? This is one way that we experience the influence of epidemiology on our work.

Coggon *et al.* (2003: 1) define epidemiology as 'the study of how often diseases occur in different groups of people and why'. Therefore epidemiology can tell us

- which groups are more at risk of ill health
- what might cause certain groups to suffer more ill health than other groups
- which groups we should target with public health initiatives to reduce morbidity.

Epidemiology can also tell us about inequalities in health when we explore the health status of vulnerable groups such as our clients. This information may highlight areas of unmet needs which can then become the focus of interventions.

What epidemiology tells us in general is that physical health has become an increasing concern in mental health. The UK National Psychiatric Morbidity Survey showed high levels of physical ill health and higher rates of death among those with mental health problems compared to the rest of the population (DH 1999b). Indeed, such are the consequences of physical ill health in our clients that Allebeck (1989) suggests that schizophrenia itself is a life shortening disease.

Epidemiology has a significant impact on our practice in the guise of public health. We should all know the prevalence of mental illness in our society is 1:4 – one in four people has at least one mental, neurological or behavioural disorder but most of these disorders are neither diagnosed nor treated (WHO 2008a). Other statistics include the following:

- The prevalence of depression is estimated at 5–10 per cent of the population at any given time (WHO 2001).
- The prevalence of schizophrenia is between 0.5 per cent and 1 per cent (Murray 2005).
- The prevalence of bipolar disorder is approximately 1 per cent of the population (NICE 2006: 76).

What is public health?

Public health is the science and art of promoting health, preventing disease and prolonging life through the organized efforts of society (WHO 1998: 3). The 'science' is represented by both epidemiology, which can track patterns of health and illness, and evidence based practice, which is employed to promote health or reduce illness. The 'art' is mental health nursing; how our interventions can prevent mental illness and prolong life, e.g. suicide prevention and promoting positive mental health. A significant new challenge is incorporating physical health into our role in respect to preventing physical conditions and promoting physical well-being.

Box 2.2 **Exercise**	How would you define incidence and prevalence? Illustrate this with reference to your current client group.

Defining some key public health concepts

Here we will explore key epidemiological concepts that can assist practitioners in implementing the physical health agenda in their settings. Whether it is inpatient acute care, long term rehabilitation or community mental health, a basic knowledge of these key concepts will enable you to focus on areas of greatest health need. This effective targeting of resources promotes evidence based practice enabling practitioners to effectively commission or advocate for physical health care services on behalf of their client group.

Demographics

Demographics is the study of human populations with regard to their current characteristics and short term trends. In general it is a particular aspect of the information collected every day and can relate to the following areas of health:

- Personal details: name, next of kin/nearest relative, address, date of birth, hospital number
- Biographical details: age, gender, ethnicity, employment status, religion, educational level
- Social details: carer address/next of kin, GP address, other relevant contacts, e.g. social worker, probation officer, benefits status, housing status
- Medical history: past medical history, current medical history, current medication, adverse drug reactions

Box 2.3   Describe the demographic profile of your client group.
Exercise

Health statistics

'Illness' and 'health' statistics are collected in many ways. Each of these acts as a barometer to the health of our clients and gives an idea of which groups, or problems, will require attention. Normally the most pertinent ones for practitioners refer to mental health care, for example, the prevalence of schizophrenia or the incidence of self harm in young people. However, what is becoming more apparent is the incidence and prevalence of physical illness in clients and more so, the high death rates for physical illness discussed in Chapter 1.

Health statistics are usually expressed as rates, that is, they indicate the frequency of something occurring. Rates can be expressed in a general way, referred to as crude rates, or they will be more specific, where they relate to specific groups within the population. For example, the rate of schizophrenia in the general population is 1:100. This means that for every 100 people, at least 1 will have schizophrenia. However, what is obvious about taking the rate is that it does not tell us how severe the schizophrenia is. Therefore rates only indicate frequency, not necessarily severity. Nevertheless, rates are important as they can give us information on how our services should be developed, or the training that practitioners may need, or the possible impact on carers. This part of the chapter will explore some useful types of statistics and illustrate how they can be used in our practice.

Figure 2.1 illustrates the prevalence of physical conditions in the general population and people with severe mental illness (SMI). It is clear that there are glaring differences in the frequency of conditions between the groups. The DRC (2006) also found that not only are people with SMI more likely to become ill, they are more likely to have poorer outcomes than those in the general population:

- People with learning disabilities or SMI die 5–10 years younger than the general population.
- Women with schizophrenia are 42 per cent more likely to get breast cancer.
- People with schizophrenia are nearly twice as likely to get bowel cancer (the second most common cause of cancer death in the UK).
- There is poor prognosis with physical illness: 22 per cent of people with CHD who have schizophrenia have died, compared with 8 per cent of people with no SMI.

The two most common rates that we have heard of are incidence rate (IR) and prevalence rate (PR). Remember the exercise at the start of the chapter? Compare your definitions of incidence and prevalence to those given below.

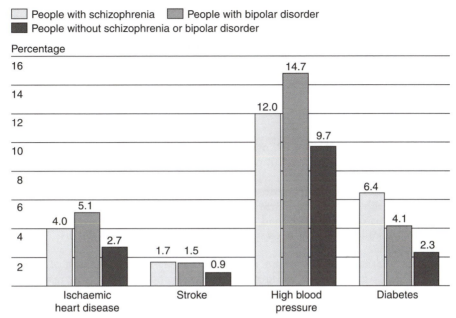

Figure 2.1 The prevalence of physical health conditions in people with schizophrenia and bipolar disorder

Source: Disability Rights Commission (DRC) (2006) reproduced with permission of the Commission for Equality and Human Rights

Note: These figures are similar to those found internationally.

Incidence

Incidence is a measure of the number of *new cases* of a condition in a defined population in a specified time. Incidence describes the frequency with which new cases of a condition are diagnosed.

Box 2.4 Case example

Simon is a community mental health nurse who wants to examine the incidence of T2D in his current caseload. In January 2008 Simon found that four people on his caseload of 30 have a diagnosis of T2D. When the same group are screened six months later the total number of people with T2D is now eight. Simon already knows that there are four confirmed cases of T2D so only 26 were at risk of developing it. Therefore the incidence is $4/26 \times 100 = 15$ per cent. The incidence of T2D in Simon's caseload is 15 per cent.

Prevalence

Prevalence is a measure of the number of *all known cases* of disease in a specific group. This can be calculated as a point prevalence – the number of known cases at a certain point of time; or as a period prevalence – the number of known cases in a certain period of time, e.g. one year. In general terms it is estimated that the prevalence of diabetes in people with schizophrenia can be 2 to 4 times higher than in the general population (Expert Consensus Group 2003).

Box 2.5 Case example

The prevalence of T2D in Simon's caseload is calculated as – all known cases of T2D (n = 8) divided by the total population at risk (n = 30); 8/30 × 100 per cent = 27 per cent. So the prevalence of T2D in Simon's caseload is 27 per cent.

Mortality rate

The mortality rate (MR) can tell us a lot about the health of the general population and of specific groups within it. The MR will not only tell us the number of deaths, it can also tell us the number of deaths between groups, for example, men and women, social classes or of different causes of death. The MR that we most associate with mental illness is the suicide rate. However, with physical illness being so prevalent, we now know that deaths from physical conditions can be higher than those from suicide. Given the high rates of deaths from physical conditions we will need to ensure that we are tackling deaths from all causes and not just suicide.

We can be more specific about the MR by calculating the number of deaths in specific populations, e.g. the risk of mortality from coronary heart disease is increased in people with severe mental illness in the 18–75 years age group (Osborn *et al.* 2007). When looking at MR it is worth considering problems associated with, for example, cause of death. If there is an error in recording cause of death or cause of death is misdiagnosed then this will affect the quality of statistics through under-reporting. Sometimes for a cause of death to be established a post-mortem may be needed and this may not often be done, apart from deaths in suspicious circumstances.

Standardized mortality ratio

The standardized mortality ratio (SMR) is the ratio of the actual number of deaths in a population to the number of deaths expected if the death rate was the same as the general population. The SMR uses 100 as a standard figure for the whole population. This signifies a national 'average' if all things were equal; it does not signify age. A figure over 100 is worse than the national average and a figure less than 100 is better. It is a good simple measure to compare areas of a country, groups within society or international comparisons at a point in time.

Let's put the SMR into perspective for our clients. Research by Harris and Barraclough (1998) shows that people with SMI have higher SMRs than the UK general population in a range of conditions:

• Cardiovascular disease SMR 250
• Respiratory disease SMR 250
• Infectious disease SMR 500

This means that our clients will die 2.5 times more often from cardiovascular disease and respiratory disorders and five times more often from infections than the general population. Again the irony here is that in many cases, clients may be in contact with healthcare services, yet their physical health needs may not be adequately addressed. These SMR statistics emphasize why we should be focusing on the physical health of clients. With such disparate death rates practitioners should be prioritizing the assessment and screening of these types of conditions so that they can be detected early and prompt interventions given.

Life expectancy

Life expectancy (LE) is the average number of years a person will live before they die. In the UK the LE for men and women has continued to rise. At birth the LE for females born in the UK was 81 years, compared with 76 years for males (ONS 2004). However, if we look at the LE for our clients we can see that it is much worse than that of the general population. Farnam *et al.* (1999) state that people with SMI have a higher risk of preventable death, estimating that this group dies between 10 to 15 years earlier than the general population.

Morbidity rate

The morbidity rate is a measure of the *frequency* of an illness or condition in the population. Be careful not to confuse mortality and morbidity, as morbidity measures the rate of illness and not the rate of death. For example, there are high rates of medical co-morbidity in our client group, especially in schizophrenia. The Disability Rights Commission (2006) found that 31 per cent of people with schizophrenia and CHD are diagnosed under 55, compared with 18 per cent of others with CHD. The late detection of conditions such as heart disease and diabetes means that our clients not only have worse MRs than the general population, but the severity of morbidity is probably greater also.

Risk

> **Box 2.6 Exercise**
>
> List the risk factors for CHD in your client group? Which of these are modifiable and which are non-modifiable?

In epidemiology risk relates to two things: the risk of developing an illness, or the risk that a particular intervention will work or not. As in mental health care there are many *risk factors* for certain conditions. A risk factor is something that can positively contribute to the risk event. For example, smoking (risk factor) can lead to lung cancer (risk event); poor diet (risk factor) can lead to a heart attack (risk event); or lack of exercise (risk factor) can lead to diabetes (risk event). From these three crude examples we can see the complex nature of relationships between risk factors and risk events. Will a lack of exercise alone lead to diabetes if the individual has a well balanced diet? What part does genetics play in this? We can also see that risk factors may not only be active (smoking) but also passive (not exercising).

Risk factors for physical illness

Risk factors can be dynamic or static; that is some are open to change, while some are not. Lifestyle factors are dynamic as with health education and promotion they can be modified, for example, smoking cessation therapy can reduce/eliminate smoking. Some risk factors are static; they are un-modifiable as health education or promotion cannot change them, for example, a genetic predisposition to an illness.

Risk factors for physical illness in our clients are the same as for the general population. It may be that the relationship between physical illness and mental illness presents us with an added level of complexity, but in general the risk factors are the same: sedentary lifestyle, poor diet, lack of exercise and smoking. A unique factor for our clients is psychotropic medication and the risk factors that this presents. This will be explored later in the book.

Exposure to risk factors

People with SMI have higher rates of physical illness than the general population which largely goes undetected (Brown *et al.* 1999). While many individuals are in contact with mental health or primary care services, the focus of interventions and interactions is naturally the primary psychiatric illness. If there is significant concern regarding physical health this will either be managed 'in house', or, depending on the severity or results from diagnostic testing, referred to either primary care services or acute/community hospital services.

When exploring illness we need to examine risk factors that can increase the risk of developing a physical condition. I am sure that you are aware of a range of risk factors that can lead to lung cancer. The most prominent one is smoking. However, there are some people who do not smoke that develop lung cancer. How can we explain this? One way is by examining their exposure to the risk factor. Therefore, while we might have an idea that people with mental illness smoke a lot, research indicates that the prevalence of smoking in people with SMI is significantly higher than that of the general population (McNeill 2001). If we explore this further we find that the rates of smoking are higher in individuals with psychotic disorders with some studies showing a prevalence of up to 80 per cent (McNeill 2001).

Our clients face increased exposure to a range of risk factors and physical illness. However, exposure to risk factors cuts two ways. While it is recognized that lifestyle factors account for some of the exposure to physical illness, the failure of health services to respond equally to clients' physical complaints also exposes them to increased risk.

For example, in comparing the impact of different risk factors on the physical health of clients we find that:

- Lifestyle factors:
  - Smoking rates are higher in individuals with psychotic disorders (McNeill 2001).
  - 33 per cent of people with schizophrenia are obese compared to 21 per cent of the general population.
- Health organization factors:
  - People with schizophrenia and stroke were less likely than the general population to have a cholesterol test.
  - 63 per cent of eligible women with schizophrenia had a cervical smear compared to 73 per cent of women in the general population (DRC 2006).

While lifestyle factors may contribute to the cause of illness, failure to respond or intervene promptly, to modify lifestyle factors or identify illness early, might be the reasons that individuals go on to develop long term morbidity or early mortality.

Table 2.1 outlines risk factors for CHD. Social class has been categorized as non-modifiable for clients as social mobility for this group is hugely restricted due to stigma and social exclusion. The challenge for us is to replicate these categories of risk factors for the different conditions present in our clients.

What does this mean for our clients?

If these statistics are ignored then it means that the current dire picture of deaths and illness from treatable physical conditions will remain unchanged. Clients and carers will face the added burden of a co-morbid physical condition and a major mental health problem. However, if the nettle is grasped, these statistics challenge us to turn the tide of ill health in our client group. Now that we know the major areas of concern – obesity, diabetes, cardiovascular illness, respiratory illness and infections – we should really begin to integrate other national service

Table 2.1 Modifiable and non-modifiable risk factors for CHD

Non-modifiable risk factors	Modifiable risk factors
Genetics	Smoking
Age	Hypertension
Gender	Lack of exercise
Ethnicity	Obesity
Family history of CHD	Anxiety/stress
Diabetes	Alcohol intake
Social class	High cholesterol
Side effects of anti-psychotic medication	
Mental illness diagnosis	

frameworks such as that for CHD (DH 2000b) and the various NICE guidance into our work routine, at least at a level of screening and onward referral.

Putting these statistics to use

A common concern of practitioners is what do we do with these statistics; how do we put them to good use? The first point would be to ensure that the statistics are collected in the first instance. Without these there will be no way of knowing what the main health problems are or how to prioritize resources. Nevertheless we already have a general idea of the areas of concern but in order to effectively prioritize resources or commission services, we need to generate our own evidence regarding the prevalence of conditions. This is called health needs assessment.

Health needs assessment

As physical health is a neglected area in mental health care, it might be safe to say that we may not have a true picture of our clients' physical care needs, unless they have a current condition. It is important that the physical health needs of clients are defined in partnership with the service user and not just left to professional opinion alone. Bradshaw's (1972) definition of need is one of the best known ways of defining need and comprises four areas:

- Normative need: needs based on criteria as set by experts or officials, e.g. the number of beds needed for a population
- Felt need: the needs as wanted by the individual
- Expressed need: the needs that the individual expresses or demands themselves
- Comparative need: based on the needs when two groups are compared

Defining needs is complex as there will be tension between what policy makers, professionals and service users define as a need. It is disempowering for clients to have their needs diminished by diagnostic overshadowing (see Chapter 1) or to have them remain as unmet because mental health nurses or services are not up to the challenge of the physical health agenda. However, it should be recognized that needs might be identified but interventions not wanted, for example, clients that smoke may not want interventions such as smoking cessation. Health needs are relative to the individual and we may have a system of bargaining our health, e.g. being a social smoker – we know smoking is bad for us but we minimize the extent that we do it.

| **Box 2.7** | What are the most prevalent physical health problems in your client group? Would |
| **Exercise** | your client group agree with you? |

Caseload profiling

Twinn *et al.* (1996) define caseload profiling as the analysis of all individual records held by each community health care nurse. However, this is not to say that our ward based records do not need profiling at regular intervals. Profiling caseloads is important as it will help us to get an accurate picture of the physical health status of our clients. It will not only help us to estimate the prevalence of physical illness but also help us to identify unmet needs which need to be highlighted. Unmet needs are not only confined to client health but also include aspects such as areas to strengthen commissioning of physical health care, equipment for assessing and maintaining physical health and staff training needs.

Table 2.2 is an example of a caseload profile. This should be preformed against each of our client's case notes. There may be obvious categorical differences in respect to what is measured. Local discussion and client or carer input will fine tune any tool.

Screening for physical conditions in clients

Caseload profiling requires us to have various clinical skills and theoretical knowledge, for example, therapeutic blood glucose levels, normal ranges for baseline observations. These procedures contribute to the process of screening which is defined as 'the application of a special test for everyone at risk of a particular disease to detect whether the disease is present at an early stage' (Ewles 2005: 283). Screening and assessment will be covered in more detail in the forthcoming chapters.

Potential benefits of health needs assessment

The benefits of health needs assessment speak for themselves: improved profiling can lead to more accurate prevalence statistics which can lead to more effective targeting of resources and interventions. Better statistics can also lead to better commissioning to underpin and support the physical health agenda. Clients can feel that their physical health is incorporated into a holistic nursing assessment. Advantages and disadvantages of health needs assessment are outlined in Table 2.3.

The challenge for MHNs – meeting the physical health needs of clients

Box 2.8 Case example

Staff nurse Ncube is increasingly concerned at the increasing weight gain in her client group. She brings this up at one of the staff meetings and it is agreed that, to help weight reduction, saccharine sweeteners will now be used on the ward rather than sugar.

As discussed previously, we need to have an idea of our clients' health beliefs. This will enable us to more effectively collaborate on determining health needs. While we know that factors such as increased calorie intake and lack of exercise can increase weight, we cannot afford to be

Table 2.2 Example of a caseload profile

Demographic breakdown	Gender Ethnicity Age Social class Psychiatric diagnosis
Respiratory health	Number of smokers Degree of tobacco use – light, moderate, heavy Prevalence of respiratory disorders – asthma, chronic obstructive pulmonary disease (COPD) Current treatment regimes Smoking cessation
Cardiovascular health	Number of people with cardiovascular problems Severity of problems Current treatment regimes
Substance misuse	Number of alcohol users Degree of alcohol use by policy defined units Prevalence of alcohol related disorders Number of substance users Degree of substance Type of substance use Mode of substance use Prevalence of associated disorders HIV/AIDS, Hep C
Nutritional status	Prevalence of overweight/obesity Degree of overweight/obesity as measured by BMI, waist-hip ratio, waist circumference Prevalence of diabetes by type Prevalence of metabolic syndrome Pre-diabetes? Current treatment for diabetes Complications of diabetes
Social factors	Benefits Social support Housing Debt/poverty/hardship Leisure
Screening/prevention	Breast screening Cervical smear Testicular screening Immunizations/vaccinations Sex education Family planning Healthy eating/dietary advice Exercise

evangelical about interventions as clients may be put off by this. Individuals may know what the message is but may not yet be at the stage where they want to change and we cannot enforce change on clients. While staff nurse Ncube's intentions may be honourable they seem very paternalistic as she is taking a well meaning decision *on behalf* of her clients. This diminishes their autonomy and ability to make decisions. This decision also limits the intervention to

Table 2.3 Possible advantages and disadvantages of health needs assessment

Advantages	Disadvantages
Accurate local health needs to inform target setting	Services and interventions rationed to specific areas
Better statistics for more appropriate commissioning	Needs classified as 'unmet' as few resources for commissioning available
Improved services/access to service	No extra resources means redistribution of mental health budgets which are already low
Improved physical health of clients	Whose responsibility is it for improving physical health – mental health services or primary care services?
Improved practitioner knowledge, skills and practice	Practitioners may not see this as part of their role and may not be confident in extending their scope of practice

lifestyle and does not include either social factors that might impact on weight gain, nor associated adverse drug reactions. Therefore while the plan – to reduce weight gain – is positive the intervention – banning sugar and using sweeteners is ill thought through.

Conclusion

This chapter has outlined the importance of having knowledge of basic concepts in epidemiology. It also explored the real-life impact of these concepts on the physical health of clients thus laying down a challenge for practitioners to employ holistic assessments in our work. It introduced the concept of health needs assessment and illustrates how it may be used in practice. However, practitioners must be cautious with using epidemiological data in the planning and delivery of health services or health interventions. While this might be seen as effective targeting of resources by some, it may be interpreted by others as rationing health services or interventions. This principle of the greater good – doing something that benefits many – is a core principle of public health as policies are directed towards the biggest killers of the population, i.e. cancer, diabetes and CHD. But what if a client's illness or condition is rare or difficult to measure epidemiologically? Finding oneself outside of the policies or interventions can be a frightening experience. Described as a post-code lottery – not being able to get treatment because your health authority/provider wants to focus on more substantial issues – means that we may need to undertake an advocacy role to ensure that clients' physical health needs, or access to treatments, are not diminished.

Summary of key points

- Long term chronic and severe physical illness are more prevalent in clients than in the general population.
- It is important that practitioners have an understanding of key terms in epidemiology so that they can assess the health needs of their clients.
- While knowledge of key terms in epidemiology is important, the challenge is to do something effective with the statistics.
- Thorough health needs assessment can lead to more effective commissioning of physical health care services for clients.

- Practitioners need to develop skills in public health techniques such as screening, physical health education and health promotion.

Quick quiz

1 In relation to your client group, list the health information that you collect.
2 How do you think this information could be put to use?
3 What are the local barriers you can identify to putting health information to use?
4 How would you begin building a physical health profile of your client group?
5 What is the prevalence of smoking in your current client caseload?

---

3 Clinical skills for physical assessment in mental health settings

By the end of this chapter you will have:

- Examined clinical governance and infection control

- Defined homeostasis

- Examined clinical observations such as temperature, pulse, blood pressure, ECG, pulse oximetry, respiration, collecting a sputum sample, peak flow, urinalysis, BMI, testing blood glucose, pathology tests for bloods

- Explored the relevance of observations in relation to mental health care

- Explored the process of care planning for some physical conditions

Box 3.1
Exercise

Which skills do you consider important for physical assessment?

Introduction

This chapter will explore the clinical skills required for examining and monitoring clients' physical health. Clinical skills are an important component of the nurse's work and those discussed here are required either for direct observation, e.g. temperature, pulse and blood pressure, or for collecting various clinical samples for testing. Testing samples can be done on the ward, e.g. urinalysis, or sent to a pathology lab, e.g. a sputum sample.

The principles of infection control are important requirements when undertaking clinical observations. All local policies and procedures pertaining to the collection, handling and safe disposal of clinical waste should be followed conscientiously by practitioners. This is important in protecting the health and safety of both clients and staff.

When performing clinical observations or taking clinical samples, hand hygiene is very important. Practitioners should wash their hands and/or use alcohol hand rub before and after contact with clients. This will minimize the chances of cross infection while increasing client confidence and reassurance that infection control is taken seriously. Practitioners should also remember the practical aspects of physical assessment outlined in Chapter 2 when undertaking clinical observations.

Clinical governance

Clinical governance is defined as 'an umbrella term for everything that helps to maintain and improve high standards of patient care' (Currie *et al.* 2003: 7). There are a range of observations used in physical assessment that we are trained to perform. However, there are risks involved in physical assessment and although small, they require management. Risks range from cross infection when using, or disposing of, clinical hazards to forgetting to perform, or document, a clinical observation. Clinical governance is the process of achieving high quality care through managing these risks.

Examples of clinical governance initiatives that manage risk and promote client safety include:

- Following established policies and procedures, e.g. infection control
- Developing and implementing clinical standards, e.g. physical assessment protocols
- Implementing clinical audit, e.g. auditing the effectiveness of physical assessment protocols
- Implementing evidence based practice, e.g. diabetes screening
- Clinical audit, e.g. evaluating the effectiveness of protocols
- Staff education and training, e.g. clinical skills refresher courses for all practitioners
- Accurate and consistent documentation and record keeping

It is important that organizations have an infrastructure in place to support physical health and well-being. This includes assessment protocols, equipment, resources and education and training. Investment in training and education is required as research by Nash (2005) shows that mental health nurses are highly motivated to undertake training in physical care skills.

**Box 3.2
Exercise**   Define homeostasis.

This chapter will illustrate clinical observation skills within a mental health specific context. The framework for physical assessment is outlined in Figure 3.1. The first two steps have been covered in depth in previous chapters and are the first two steps in assessing the physical health of clients. The general survey will tell us general information; the physical assessment will support our general survey findings; and the clinical observations will corroborate our findings and confirm whether or not further investigations are warranted.

While there are a wide range of clinical observations those that will be covered in this chapter include:

- Temperature
- Pulse
- Blood pressure
- Electrocardiogram
- Pulse oximetry
- Respiration rate
- Collecting a sputum sample
- Peak flow
- Urinalysis
- Body mass index
- Testing blood glucose
- Pathology tests for bloods

The rationale for selecting these is that they are the key observations associated with the prevalent physical illnesses outlined in this book. Other clinical skills are undertaken by more appropriately qualified nurses, e.g. a diabetic leg ulcer assessment will be undertaken by a tissue viability nurse or diabetes nurse specialist. However, skills can be taught and it is important that

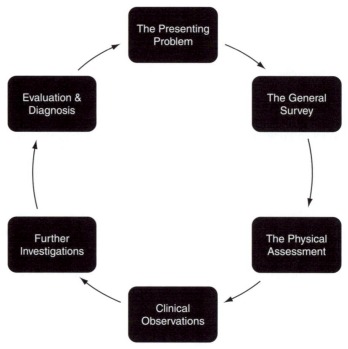

Figure 3.1 The process of physical assessment and observation

our repertoire of skills in physical care grows. This can be reflected in our post-registration education where we may opt for courses in physical health such as tissue viability.

The key techniques in physical assessment are

- observation
- palpation
- inspection
- auscultation

Rationale for taking baseline observations

Baseline observations are an essential part of the physical assessment of an existing condition or the monitoring of an established one. These observations provide clinically important data such as

- baseline measurements for future comparison
- screening for previously undiagnosed conditions
- monitoring previously diagnosed illnesses
- determining the response to treatment of a current physical illness
- monitoring the course of a current physical condition(s)
- promoting early intervention
- selecting the best intervention or treatment

When undertaking clinical observations you should endeavour to protect the client's privacy and dignity.

Homeostasis

Homeostasis is the regulation by an organism of the chemical composition of its body fluids and other aspects of its internal environment so that physiological processes can proceed at optimum rates (*Oxford Dictionary of Biology*, 4th edition, 2000). In homeostasis a system will make adjustments to restore balance when there is interruption from internal and external disturbances.

Components of a homeostatic system

A homeostatic system has four components (see Figure 3.2).

- The control centre sets the predetermined reference points for homeostasis, e.g. body temperature, pulse rate or insulin levels.
- A receptor detects changes that cause a homeostatic imbalance. It sends a message to the control centre outlining this.
- The control centre sends a message to an effector to act and restore homeostasis, e.g. a message goes to the pancreas to release more insulin.
- A feedback loop – the effector sends a message to the control centre confirming action and the control centre responds when homeostatic balance has been regained.

Homeostasis controls a range of clinical observations e.g. pulse, blood pressure and glucose/insulin release. We can illustrate homeostasis with reference to temperature as in Table 3.1.

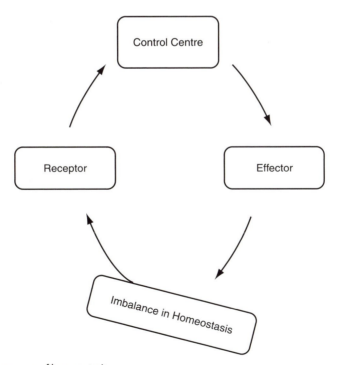

Figure 3.2 The process of homeostasis

Table 3.1 The homeostasis of body temperature

System	Function	Example
1 Reference point	The predetermined level at which the body is in homeostasis.	Temperature between 36.0°C–37.2°C.
2 Receptor	This is a sensor that responds to changes in the environment that may put homeostasis into imbalance.	Thermoreceptors in the skin and blood pick up an increase in temperature. They send a message confirming this to the control centre.
3 Control centre (Hypothalamus)	This sets the range of values for reference points. The control centre monitors and evaluates all information to maintain homeostasis.	The control centre senses that the body temperature is rising over its pre-determined level so sends messages to mechanisms involved in temperature control, e.g. the skin, sweat glands, blood vessels and cells, endocrine system.
4 Effector	This receives messages from the control centre when there is imbalance. The effector will produce a response that restores homeostasis.	The skin starts to sweat to lose heat, blood vessels dilate to lose heat. If increase in temperature is due to infection white blood cells are sent to fight infection, the endocrine systems slows metabolism to prevent more heat being generated until temperature returns to normal.
5 A feedback loop	The effector sends a message back to the control centre.	The message confirms that homeostasis has been restored and the effector can stop.

Homeostasis is a good concept for guiding the nursing process:

- Assessment – body temperature is out of balance
- Diagnosis – client is pyrexic
- Plan – restore homeostasis
- Implement – interventions to restore normal temperature
- Evaluate – has homeostasis been restored?

Box 3.3 Exercise Outline the infection control issues that need consideration when undertaking a physical assessment.

Observation

Assessing physical health is an important skill given the prevalence of physical conditions in our client group. Factors that will influence assessment include the approach you use and the presenting complaint. Therefore it is very important that you know your client, their past medical history and any significant close family history of physical illness.

Box 3.4 Case example

Simon has been admitted to your ward following a crisis visit. He has a history of schizo-affective disorder. He is presenting in an agitated and anxious state. Staff are putting his physical presentation down to his not wanting to be admitted and his anxiety at leaving home. He is refusing any interaction with staff preferring to have a cigarette alone. A little while later you notice Simon is more subdued but he has breathing difficulties and is clutching his chest. From observation alone we can make a quick assessment.

Assessment

General appearance – Simon appears to be physically unwell, skin is ashen colour, he is sweaty and lips are cyanosed, oedema evident in ankles, hands cold to touch

Lifestyle risk factors – smoking

Respiration – audible breathing distress, rapid and shallow breaths, experiences chest pain (client clasps chest)

Mobility – normally fine but now is immobile, when trying to move he expends a lot of effort

Baseline observations

Blood pressure = 180/100, Pulse 140, Respirations 22 shallow and rapid, Temperature 38.2°C

Diagnosis

Suspected myocardial infarction or heart failure

Plan

Activate medical emergency and transfer to acute care or accident and emergency services.

Observation is an important skill as at times it will indicate the nature of the presenting complaint as an emergency (as illustrated in Box 3.4) or as routine screening. Observation needs to be quick and effective. Even in the unlikely event that Simon turns out to have severe indigestion, you will not be faulted for suspecting something more sinister. Indeed at times the reverse is true; the sinister complaint is ignored due to the client's mental health problem. Observation is a valuable skill when clients do not consent to a physical exam, as a crude assessment can be made from a distance (see Chapter 4). Nevertheless, we must have the prerequisite knowledge and skills in physical health to make use of observation skills. We should always confirm our observations with a clinical assessment.

Clinical skills used routinely in mental health care

Temperature

Temperature is one of the core clinical observations. Our body temperature is regulated by the thermo-regulatory centre of the hypothalamus. The temperature observation can either be too low or too high.

Table 3.2 Temperature ranges

Temperature	Range
Hypothermia	Below 35°C
Normal Temperature range	36.0°C–37.2°C
Pyrexia	Greater than 37.5°C
• Low Grade Pyrexia	36.7°C–38°C
• Moderate – High Grade Pyrexia	38°C–40°C
Hyper-pyrexia	Greater than 40°C

Source: Adapted from Mains *et al.* (2008)

Taking a temperature reading

The first point in taking a temperature is determining the site to obtain a reading, e.g. orally, from the forehead or from the ear canal. These sites are less invasive and do not require disrobing. The axilla (under arm) site is also used but this is a little more invasive as disrobing may be required. In cases of hypothermia a rectal temperature is required. When documenting the temperature reading, you should indicate the site used.

Equipment

There are two types of thermometer, digital and non-digital. Both types are used to take readings from various sites. A tympanic thermometer works by using an infra-red light to detect heat rising from the tympanic membrane providing a digital reading (Nicol *et al.* 2004). A non-digital thermometer, e.g. Tempadot, can be used to take oral or axilla readings. It is important that the correct equipment is used when taking the temperature reading, e.g. an oral thermometer should not be used for a rectal temperature.

Infection control and equipment issues

Whichever equipment is used the principles of infection control should be followed to prevent risk of cross infection. Single use only devices should be used and new tympanic covers employed each time a new temperature recording is required.

Although more convenient to use, tympanic thermometers require careful handling and use under manufacturer's recommendations. They also need regular servicing to ensure they are fit for purpose. You should be aware of instructions for use as a variety, from a range of manufacturers, may be in use. For example, some tympanic thermometers have a single use facility where it will not function unless a new cap is put on. Some tympanic thermometers have memory functions so it is important that what you record is the real time reading and not one stored in the memory. Batteries will also require frequent review to ensure they are well charged.

Procedure for taking a temperature reading

Here we focus on taking an oral temperature reading with a non-digital thermometer (see Table 3.3). If taking a temperature reading via axilla, irrespective of thermometer type, you should respect the client's privacy and dignity.

Table 3.3 Taking an oral temperature reading with a non-digital thermometer

Step	Action	Rationale
1 Prepare equipment	Select thermometer, pen, chart for recording result	To ensure effective monitoring and prompt recording of reading
2 Decontaminate hands	Wash hands or use alcohol rub	To promote infection control and minimise cross infection
3 Explain procedure	Outline your intended actions	To reassure the client and gain consent
4 Ensure client is rested and relaxed	Ensure client has not smoked or drunk tea/coffee beforehand	To minimize biased readings
5 Ask client to open their mouth	Insert the thermometer under the tongue	This will give a reading that is close to the core body temperature
6 Ask the client to close their mouth	Advise the client to envelop the thermometer when their mouth is closed. Advise them not to bite or chew on the thermometer. Refrain from talking until the procedure is over	Enveloping the thermometer will prevent air from impairing the reading. Biting and chewing will ruin the thermometer and may cause small cuts. Talking will allow air into the oral cavity which will reduce the accuracy of the reading
7 Leave the thermometer for one minute	As above	This will give enough time to get an accurate reading. If pulse recording is also required it may be done within this time also
8 Remove thermometer	Ensure you do not touch the exposed part	To prevent exposure to potential infection
9 Record and document your findings	Ensure you are familiar with the standard way to record depending on the type of thermometer used	The appropriate chart should be completed accurately for comparison with other past, or for future readings
10 Communicate findings 1	Inform client of the outcome and be prepared to answer any queries they may have	To reassure the client
11 Communicate findings 2	Report any abnormalities to the nurse in charge	In case immediate intervention is required or for continuity of care
12 Communicate findings 3	Record findings in the client's case notes	So that other members of the team are aware of them
13 Decontaminate hands again	Wash hands or use alcohol rub	To promote infection control and minimize cross infection

Box 3.5 Case example

Michael is a 38-year-old male with a history of psychotic disorder. He is currently receiving risperidone 3mg twice daily. He smokes thirty cigarettes daily and takes little exercise. He reports not feeling well over the last few days. You take his observations and find that his temperature is 38.6°. What do you do?

Assessment

Michael has a temperature of 38.6°. He feels unwell and has a cough that is producing greenish sputum.

Diagnosis

Michael has a chest infection as he has a fever and his temperature homeostasis is out of balance. Reasons for this include:

- Michael is pyrexic, he has a productive cough, sputum is greenish in colour.
- Michael is a smoker and is more vulnerable to chest infections.
- Michael has probably contracted influenza.
- Michael is also taking an anti-psychotic medication that may cause blood irregularities.

Plan

Return Michael's temperature to normal homeostatic balance. An inter-professional approach will be required involving Michael's doctor. Baseline observations indicate fever so more information regarding the nature of the suspect infection is required.

- Blood tests for pathology are required to determine the exact nature of the infection and antibiotic to prescribe – full blood count including white cell count.
- Infection may be due to low white cell count as an adverse drug reaction.
- Collect a sputum sample for pathology.

Implementation

Pathology tests indicate a chest infection. An adverse drug reaction has been excluded from the diagnosis. After a team discussion it is decided Michael requires a course of antibiotics.

- Take Michael's baseline observations two hourly for the first 48 hours then four hourly thereafter until homeostasis returns. Remember the principles of infection control to prevent cross infection.
- Ensure Michael complies with antibiotic medications. Monitoring should be for desired and undesired effects of the treatment.
- Encourage Michael to reduce smoking to promote recuperation.
- Encourage Michael to bed rest as much as possible but also ensure mobility to maintain independence. Advise Michael that he may feel generally weak and may be unsteady so he should mobilize with care to prevent falling.
- Encourage Michael to dress appropriately to avoid becoming overly cold or hot.
- Encourage Michael to sit upright to ensure he can clear any sputum.
- Encourage Michael to use hankies and to cover his mouth when coughing and sneezing to minimize cross infection.
- Encourage adequate fluid balance to prevent dehydration.
- Ensure Michael has adequate pillows for proper positioning at night time.
- Ensure night staff are aware of the care plan to promote continuity of care.
- Regularly monitor the care plan to determine progress.

Evaluate

- Evaluate care plan at the end of each shift to determine progress. Monitor observations, fluid balance, medication compliance and smoking behaviour.
- Michael should be asked how he is feeling for a subjective evaluation of the care

plan. As temperature falls baseline observations can revert from two to four hourly.
- Evaluation will continue daily until temperature homeostasis is restored. Michael should be advised that the course of antibiotics will need to be completed even though temperature may be within normal limits.
- As Michael is in a high risk group vaccinations for influenza and pneumococcal infection should be discussed with him to minimize potential future episodes.

Pulse

Pulse is the regular, recurrent expansion and contraction of an artery produced by waves of pressure caused by the ejection of blood from the left ventricle (Anderson and Anderson 1995). The pulse can be felt wherever an artery is near the surface of the skin, passing over a bone.

Taking a pulse

The first point of taking a pulse is determining the site that the pulse is going to be measured from. Figure 3.3 outlines the main pulse points. The pulse is usually taken at the radial site (Figure 3.4) as it is accessible and does not require disrobing.

Characteristics of a 'normal' pulse

Pulse measurement assesses pulse quality and this gives an indication of heart function. The volume of blood pumped by the heart usually remains constant. Any variation in the amount of blood being pumped will result in a quicker or slower pulse. Pulse rate and blood pressure differ with age. The 'normal' pulse rate for a healthy adult is between 60 and 100 beats per minute (Lynn 2004). Rate, rhythm and amplitude are the three key components of pulse assessment (see Table 3.4).

Pulse monitoring

Pulse monitoring will be undertaken at various times, for example, when clients report being unwell. It will certainly be taken on admission for a baseline reading and depending on the quality it may be done either routinely or periodically thereafter. Routine pulse monitoring may be in response to a current physical condition that is under treatment or to monitor the side effects of medication. Recording will occur at various times, e.g. twice daily (BD) once in the morning and evening, or if it is a serious heart condition, up to four times daily (QID).

Procedure for taking a pulse

See Table 3.5 for a description of the procedure. Be careful not to put too much pressure on the pulse point as this will be uncomfortable for the client and may make the pulse harder to detect. If the pulse point is difficult to locate begin again. It is important to be relaxed to minimize unnecessary anxiety which may increase the client's heart rate and render a false pulse reading.

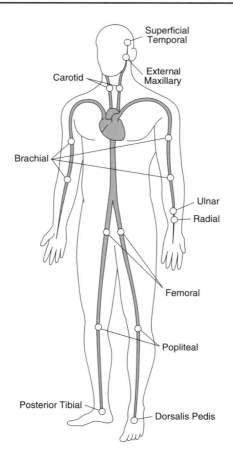

Figure 3.3 Pulse points

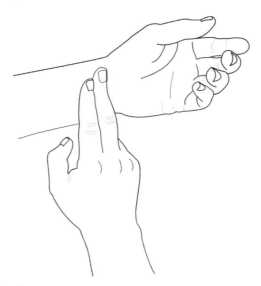

Figure 3.4 Taking a radial pulse

Table 3.4 Characteristics of the pulse

Characteristic	Definition	Abnormal
Rate	the number of times the heart beats	Under 60 and over 100 beats per minute
Rhythm	a series of regular beats	Irregular beats, missed beats
Amplitude	how long the pulse lasts for	Weak and thready or strong and bounding

Table 3.5 Procedure for taking a pulse

Step	Action	Rationale
1 Prepare equipment	Watch with a second hand, pen, chart for recording result	To ensure effective monitoring and prompt recording of reading
2 Decontaminate hands	Wash hands or use alcohol rub	To promote infection control and minimize cross infection
3 Explain procedure	Outline your intended actions	To gain consent
4 Ensure client is rested and relaxed	Rested for five minutes, has not smoked or drunk tea/coffee	To minimize biased readings
5 Place finger tips (as indicated in diagram 4)	Firmly press on the radial pulse	Too little or too much pressure may make pulse recording difficult
6 Palpate pulse	Rate, rhythm and amplitude for one minute	To get an assessment of heart function Do not measure partially then multiply, always count for 1 minute
7 Record and document your findings	Complete appropriate chart	For comparison with other past or future readings
8 Communicate findings 1	Inform client of the outcome and be prepared to answer any queries they may have	To reassure the client
9 Communicate findings 2	Report any abnormalities to the nurse in charge	In case immediate intervention is required or for continuity of care
10 Communicate findings 3	Record findings in the client's case notes	So that other members of the team are aware of them
11 Decontaminate hands again	Wash hands or use alcohol rub	To promote infection control and minimize cross infection

Box 3.6 Case example

Joe is about to be discharged home. His mental state is stable following a depressive episode and he is positive for the future. He is discharged with a prescription of SSRI antidepressants. On discharge his pulse rate is 84. What do you do?

Knowing how to interpret clinical observations is an important skill. In the example in Box 3.6 Joe's pulse is only slightly elevated. We might assume that Joe has a certain amount of anxiety about his discharge which may have increased his heart rate. We can suggest that Joe mentions this when he next goes to see his GP or his community mental health nurse so that it can be reassessed. We would record the observation and document our actions.

When clinical observations hover above or below the normal and abnormal ranges there is always a clinical decision to be made. This causes anxiety. It is easier to make clinical decisions when there is a clear cut abnormality. For example, what would your response be if Joe's pulse was 160? Obviously very different from that above, as it is a more critical situation with greater risk.

Blood pressure

Box 3.7   List the factors that can affect blood pressure readings.
Exercise

Blood pressure (BP) is defined as the pressure of blood against the walls of the main arteries (Jevon 2007a). BP is the product of cardiac output × peripheral resistance (based on Waugh and Grant 2006). The main function of maintaining BP is to ensure adequate perfusion of organs (Jevon 2007a). Without adequate blood supply organs lose their function due to tissue and cell damage, resulting in long term chronic conditions.

Equipment

The sphygmomanometer is used to measure BP. These are available in two varieties – the manual and the digital. Mercury sphygmomanometers, although still in use, are becoming less common due to the presence of mercury. If a machine is accidentally damaged and a mercury spillage ensues, this has to be cleaned at great expense. Therefore non-mercury manual sphygmomanometers are becoming more popular.

Digital sphygmomanometers are also used. These are more convenient with some also measuring pulse. However, unless kept well serviced, under manufacturers' recommended conditions they can lose calibration. This can result in mis-readings, as can low batteries or mistakenly recording measurements from the machine's memory. Digital sphygmomanometers do not require you to listen for the Korotkoff sounds but it is always good practice to do so. If you rely on this type of sphygmomanometer for pulse readings be aware that all you are getting is the rate. You are not getting the rhythm or amplitude, therefore you are missing out on two areas of pulse assessment.

'Normal' blood pressure

BP is an evaluation of how well the cardiovascular system is functioning. The standard 'normal' BP is given as 120/80 mmHg. The first number, 120 mmHg, is the systolic pressure. This is the pressure produced when the heart is active. The second number, 80 mmHg, is the diastolic pressure. When the heart is not pumping it is relaxing, allowing blood to flow in, in preparation for the next pump. This is called diastole. It is lower than the systolic pressure.

These readings may not be exactly 120/80 mmHg; they may be slightly higher (125/85 mmHg) or lower (115/75 mmHg). Therefore a range for 'normal' BP may be more appropriate. The British Heart Foundation (2005a) suggest

- Normal BP range – a blood pressure below 140/85mmHg
- If you have diabetes – a target blood pressure below 130/80mmHg

What is clear is that an increase or decrease of 30mmHg in diastolic or systolic blood pressure would be a cause of concern, more so if other risk factors for cardiovascular illness are present.

Blood pressure monitoring

Monitoring BP is similar to monitoring pulse which is outlined above.

Korotkoff sounds and blood pressure measurement

When we take a manual blood pressure reading the sounds we hear that represent a blood pressure reading are called the Korotkoff sounds. There are five phases and for the BP reading we record Phase 1 (systolic) and Phase 5 (diastolic) (see Table 3.6).

Procedure for taking a blood pressure

Table 3.7 outlines the procedure for taking blood pressure in fifteen clear stages, with the rationale for each.

Factors affecting BP readings

Sometimes BP readings will be high or low. There are two sets of circumstances that can account for this; physiological factors such as illness, or poor technique. If our technique is not up to date, our equipment not correct or proper procedures not followed, then errors in measurement will occur. Physiological factors and technique can affect blood pressure readings in the following ways:

1 *Physiological factors*
   - The stroke volume (the beating of the left ventricle)
   - Left ventricular failure
   - The elasticity of the aorta and other large arteries to distend and take the pumped blood
   - Physical conditions – aneurysm, artherosclerosis, myocardial infarction
   - Blood volume
   - Reduced blood flow following a self-harm incident
   - The viscosity (thickness) of the blood
   - Poor cardiac conduction
   - Stimulants, e.g. alcohol/smoking

2 *Technique*
   - Activity, e.g. talking/exercise immediately prior to BP
   - Clothing obstructing cuff
   - Inadequate cuff size, ill fitting cuff
   - Sphygmomanometer not calibrated or not functioning correctly
   - Eating a recent meal

Table 3.6 The Korotkoff Sounds

Korotkoff Sounds	Manifestation
Phase I	A sharp tapping
Phase 2	A swishing or whooshing sound
Phase 3	A thump softer than the tapping in phase I
Phase 4	A soft blowing muffled sound that fades
Phase 5	Silence

Source: From Kozier *et al.* (2008: 365)

Table 3.7 Procedure for taking blood pressure

Step	Action	Rationale
1 Prepare equipment	Sphygmomanometer with appropriate cuff size, pen, chart for recording result	To ensure effective monitoring and prompt recording of reading
2 Decontaminate hands	Wash hands or use alcohol rub	To promote infection control and minimize cross infection
3 Explain procedure	Outline your intended actions and warn about cuff pressure	To gain consent and prepare the client for slight discomfort
4 Ensure client is rested and relaxed	Rested for five minutes, has not smoked or drunk tea/coffee	To minimize biased readings
5 Position of patient and clothing	Upper arm is at same level of heart, clothes are not restricting cuff placement	Poor positioning and clothing obstruction may affect reading
6 Palpate pulse	Palpate radial pulse in preparation of positioning stethoscope	Proper positioning to get an accurate reading
7 Inflate cuff to 70mmHg	Note the pressure at which the pulse disappears	Correct positioning of bell of stethoscope over point of brachial artery
8 Inflate the cuff	To a further 30mmHg then point of radial pulse disappearing	To prepare to take full blood pressure reading
9 Record and document your findings	Complete appropriate chart	For comparison with other past or future readings
10 Deflate the system	Slowly and carefully so that blood pressure sounds are heard	To ensure you can hear the five phases of the Korotkoff sounds
11 Observe first and last Korotkoff Sounds	Record Korotkoff Sounds	This is the actual blood pressure
12 Communicate findings 1	Inform client of the outcome and be prepared to answer any queries they may have	To reassure the client
13 Communicate findings 2	Report any abnormalities to the nurse in charge	In case immediate intervention is required or for continuity of care
14 Communicate findings 3	Record findings in the client's case notes	So that other members of the team are aware of them
15 Decontaminate hands again	Wash hands or use alcohol rub	To promote infection control and minimise cross infection

- Emotional state – anxiety, stress; white coat effect (anxiety arising out of request for a blood pressure reading)
- Posture, e.g. poor arm positioning
- Medication given shortly before reading is taken

Electrocardiogram

The cardiac conduction system is monitored using an electrocardiogram (ECG). The ECG picks up the heart's electrical activity through pads placed on the skin in the thoracic area. The 12-lead ECG is most often used as it gives a more accurate interpretation of the rhythm than a single lead cardiac monitor (Jevon 2007b). The ECG is an important diagnostic tool and it can be used to identify a range of cardiac conditions, e.g. angina, myocardial infarction or palpitations, for example, atrial and ventricular fibrillation.

In mental health care an ECG is recommended when clients initiate and receive certain antipsychotic medications, for example, a baseline ECG is taken on commencement of clozapine and periodically thereafter. Specific adverse drug reactions can impair the cardiac conduction system (see Chapter 8) so ECG becomes a valuable test when monitoring our client's cardiac function.

Your role in ECG monitoring is likely to be determined in local policy and procedures or clinical governance standards, if they exist. However, it is safe to say that in many instances taking an ECG will be deferred to a doctor or ECG technician. This is due to a lack of training for this procedure in mental health nursing. This can impact on our confidence to learn this skill and undertake it in clinical practice. However, ECG should be within our scope of practice given the regularity of its use in monitoring adverse drug reactions. It would be worthwhile exploring how you get local training in this procedure as it would be a valuable addition to your repertoire of skills.

Recording an ECG

Using more leads means that the heart can be scrutinized from more angles; the more angles the more comprehensive the ECG.

- A three lead ECG views the heart from 3 angles.
- A five lead ECG views the heart from 7 angles.
- A twelve lead ECG views the heart from 12 angles

(Pope 2008)

Equipment

You will need a cardiac monitor, ECG leads, gauze/alcohol wipes for cleaning the skin and excess hair may need to be removed by razor. You should ensure any equipment is stored and maintained according to the manufacturer's recommendations.

The leads for ECG machines are colour-coded to help facilitate easy placement. For example in a three lead ECG:

- Red lead (right arm cable) would go to the right shoulder,
- Yellow lead (left arm cable) to the left shoulder and
- Green lead (leg lead) to the lower chest wall (Jevon 2007b).

Practical considerations

The client should be lying and as they need to disrobe it is important to preserve their privacy and dignity. Gender specific staff choices should be respected if females do not want ECGs performed by male practitioners. If this is not an issue, chaperones should be considered.

You should carefully explain the procedure and answer client questions and concerns. If the ECG is an emergency the client should be reassured and the procedure outlined to them. Continual reassurance will be important not only because the procedure may be a concern, but they may also be feeling palpitations anyway so they will be highly anxious.

Procedure

Depending on your level of practice (whether or not you are trained to perform an ECG) your role will be either primary – performing the ECG – or secondary – assisting the practitioner performing the ECG.

Procedure for taking a 3 lead ECG

Table 3.8 outlines clearly the sixteen steps in taking a 3 lead ECG, with the rationale for each.

Results

The ECG printout will show the PQRST complex (see Chapter 5). Here we can see how the heart is functioning in respect to atrial and ventricular depolarization and repolarization. If there are big variations, e.g. due to adverse drug reactions, then medication regimes may require changing to reduce the risk of serious physical harm.

Pulse oximetry

Our body cells and tissues need a continuous supply of oxygen. A compromised oxygen supply can have serious consequences, e.g. myocardial ischaemia. Pulse oximetry is a non-invasive method of monitoring how much oxygen a person has in their blood stream without the need to take blood. The pulse oximeter measures the absorption of light waves as they pass through areas of the body that are highly perfused by arterial blood (Buchfa and Fries 2004).

Pulse oximetry works on the assumption that deoxygenated and oxygenated blood are different colours and a sensor can measure this difference, calculating the percentage of oxygen in the blood (Dougherty and Lister 2008). The sensor may be placed on the patient's fingertip or earlobe. When using the ear, results will be inaccurate if the patient's earlobe is poorly perfused, e.g. from a low cardiac output (Buchfa and Fries 2004). You should not take a pulse oximetry reading from a site where a blood pressure cuff is applied as the inflation of the cuff will decrease blood supply and give a false reading.

SaO_2 is the clinical measurement for oxygen saturation levels. The normal SaO_2 levels for adults are between 95 per cent and 100 per cent (Potter and Perry 2005). Lower SaO_2 levels require further investigation. Possible reasons for low SaO_2 levels are shown in Table 3.9.

Procedure for taking a pulse oximetry reading

See Table 3.10 for a clear step-by-step outline of the stages in this procedure, complete with rationales. Pulse oximetry measures oxygenation so it will not give an indication of carbon dioxide levels, therefore arterial blood gases will be required. Haemoglobin may also be bound to something other than oxygen, e.g. in cases of attempted suicide by suffocation haemoglobin may bind to carbon monoxide.

If equipment is not responding as you believe it should, check the client's vital signs. Do not automatically assume the machine is faulty. Most importantly, ensure you have had training and that you use equipment under manufacturer's recommendations. You should also know and understand your local policy and procedures on the use of pulse oximetry. In many cases it is now used to monitor clients who have been subject to physical restraint.

Table 3.8 The sixteen steps in taking a 3-lead ECG

Steps	Actions	Rationale
1 Prepare equipment	Ensure you have cables, ensure electrode pads are in date and the machine has enough paper for recording ECG	To ensure effective monitoring and prompt recording of reading
2 Explain procedure	Outline your intended actions	To gain consent and reassure the client
3 Ensure privacy	Carry out procedure in a suitable clinical environment	To show respect and preserve dignity
4 Decontaminate hands	Wash hands or use alcohol rub	To promote infection control and minimize cross infection
5 Ensure client is rested and relaxed	Talk to the client and give reassurance	To minimize biased readings
6 Prepare skin	Ensure skin is clean and dry. Shave excess hair	To ensure the electrode has good contact with the skin
7 Place electrodes onto the selected skin areas		In preparation for connecting the leads to the monitor
8 Connect the three leads and turn on monitor	Ensure the leads connect with the colour coded inputs and select which lead the reading will be taken from	To ensure accurate assessment of heart function
9 Set any alarms on the machine	Follow local clinical standards or policy for this	Set the normal ranges so that tachycardia or bradycardia will sound. This allows you to ensure the client is not in cardiac distress. Always check the client if an alarm sounds – do not assume it is a mechanical problem.
10 Safely dispose of used equipment	Place used electrodes and cleaning materials or alcohol wipes in appropriate clinical waste bin	To ensure promote clinical hygiene and cleanliness
11 Restore equipment safely	Ensure all leads are accounted for and paper restocked if needed	In preparation for next usage
12 Record and document your findings	Complete appropriate chart	For comparison with other past or future readings
13 Communicate findings 1	Inform client of the outcome and be prepared to answer any queries they may have	To reassure the client
14 Communicate findings 2	Report any abnormalities to the nurse in charge	In case immediate intervention is required or for continuity of care
15 Communicate findings 3	Record findings in the client's case notes	So that other members of the team are aware of them
16 Decontaminate hands again	Wash hands or use alcohol rub	To promote infection control and minimize cross infection

Box 3.8 Exercise How can MHNs reduce the risks of cardiovascular disease in their client group?

Table 3.9 Factors affecting pulse oximetry readings

Clinical reasons	Procedural reasons
Hypothermia	Cold or calloused fingertip
Low cardiac output	Patient movement e.g. tremor, shivering
Hypovolaemia	Not trained to use pulse oximetry
Heavy smoker	Machine malfunction
Inadequate blood flow due to blood pressure being taken at the same time	

Table 3.10 Procedure for taking a pulse oximetry reading

Step	Action	Rationale
1 Prepare equipment	Pulse oximeter, leads and sensor, pen, chart for recording result	To ensure effective monitoring and prompt recording of reading
2 Decontaminate hands	Wash hands or use alcohol rub	To promote infection control and minimize cross infection
3 Explain procedure	Outline your intended actions and select site to attach sensor	To gain consent and prepare the client for slight discomfort
4 Ensure client is rested and relaxed	Reassure client	This may be a new experience for them and they may be anxious
5 Clean the site	Use an alcohol wipe to clean the area	Excessive dirt may give false reading, nail polish or false nails may also give false readings (Nichol *et al.* 2003)
6 Attach sensor	Clip sensor firmly to chosen site	To obtain reading
7 Record and document the measurement	Complete appropriate chart	For comparison with other past or future readings
8 Take off sensor	If intermittent readings are needed change site	To ensure skin does not become irritated. If continuous readings are required change site every four hours (Nichol *et al.* 2003)
9 Return equipment	Carefully clean and store equipment	In preparation for next usage
10 Decontaminate hands again	Wash hands or use alcohol rub	To promote infection control and minimize cross infection
11 Communicate findings 1	Inform client of the outcome and be prepared to answer any queries they may have	To reassure the client
12 Communicate findings 2	Report any abnormalities to the nurse in charge	In case immediate intervention is required or for continuity of care
13 Communicate findings 3	Record findings in the client's case notes	So that other members of the team are aware of them

Respiration

Recording respiration rate gives an assessment of the respiratory system and lung function (see Table 3.11).

Table 3.11 Respiration rates

Respiration type	Range
Bradypnoea	Below 10 respirations per minute
Normal respiration range	12–18 per minute
Tachypnoea	Above 20 respirations per minute

Table 3.12 Procedure for taking a respiration rate

Step	Action	Rationale
1 Prepare equipment	Watch with second hand, pen and chart for recording result	To ensure effective monitoring and prompt recording of reading
2 Decontaminate hands	Wash hands or use alcohol rub	To promote infection control and minimize cross infection
3 Do not explain procedure	You may ask the client for their wrist as if to take their pulse	If client knows their respirations are going to be monitored they may try to control their breathing
4 Ensure client is rested and relaxed	Ensure client has not walked or ran for five minutes before procedure	To minimize biased readings
5 While timing count each respiration the client makes	A respiration is one inspiration and one expiration	To ensure the client is breathing normally
6 Listen for any abnormal sounds	Note if you hear any wheezing or crackling	This may indicate the presence of a respiratory condition
7 Observe lips and extremities	If there are respiratory problems there may be cyanosis	If cyanosis is present this may require further and urgent investigation
8 Record and document your findings	Ensure you are familiar with the standard way to record	The appropriate chart should be completed accurately for comparison with other past, or for future readings
9 Communicate findings 1	Inform client of the outcome and be prepared to answer any queries they may have	To reassure the client
10 Communicate findings 2	Report any abnormalities to the nurse in charge	In case immediate intervention is required or for continuity of care
11 Communicate findings 3	Record findings in the client's case notes	So that other members of the team are aware of them
12 Decontaminate hands again	Wash hands or use alcohol rub	To promote infection control and minimize cross infection

Equipment

For recording respiration rate you will need a watch with a second hand.

Procedure for taking a respiration rate

See Table 3.12 for a step by step outline of this procedure, with rationale.

Collecting a sputum sample

If a client presents with cough, with or without fever, a sputum sample may be requested for pathology analysis. This will determine the presence of infection. Sputum analysis will inform clinical decision making regarding appropriate antibiotic therapy, or if further investigations, e.g. biopsy, are required. Analysis may also detect any other foreign body present in the sample, e.g. blood.

Sputum collection is usually a straightforward process of expectoration (the client coughing up sputum) which is collected in a sterile container, clearly labelled with the client details, ward address and a description of the test to be performed. This is normally written as 'culture and sensitivity'. Other collateral information may be appropriate, e.g. if pyrexic or currently taking antibiotics. For infection control purposes, the container should be secured, so the lid does not come off, and sent in a clearly labelled biohazard bag.

At times the client may find difficulty expectorating sputum as it may be painful, leading to breathlessness or increased anxiety. Chest massage may be required to loosen or 'shift' the sputum, making it easier to expel. A physiotherapist may be required to do this or they may teach staff how to perform this type of chest percussion. Following chest massage the client should be encouraged to expectorate so that a sample is obtained.

Depending on the condition a number of sputum samples may be required. It is important that a sputum sample is collected and not a sample of saliva. The client may be embarrassed at coughing up sputum so reassure and support them. Samples should not be taken directly after meals in case the coughing leads to vomiting.

Procedure for taking a sputum sample

See Table 3.13 for a clear outline of the steps involved in taking a sputum sample, with rationales. Following the procedure the client may be tired. They should be offered a warm drink to help relax and this will also help moisten the mouth and throat which may be dry following the coughing. If required they should be observed until they have settled.

Peak flow

Peak expiratory flow rate (PEFR) is defined as 'the maximum flow rate, in litres per minute that can be expelled from the lungs during a forced exhalation' (Bennett 2003a:185). The main use of peak flow is the diagnosis and monitoring of asthma, as part of an asthma management plan, assessing severity of an asthma attack and monitoring the response to asthma therapy (Booker 2007).

If one of your clients has asthma, then PEFR may be recommended on a daily basis as this can monitor the course of the condition and how well it is responding to treatment. Here the client will be given a chart where they can plot their PEFR reading. Great variations in PEFR readings may be indicative of

- the asthma being poorly managed;
- the client not taking their inhaler medication as prescribed, e.g. they may only take it in response to an attack rather than to prevent an attack;
- poor inhaler technique where clients do not get the correct dose of medication;
- poor technique in performing PEFR.

Equipment

For recording this observation you will need a PEFR meter, a clean mouth piece, a blank sheet of paper, a pen and the PEFR recording chart.

Table 3.13 Procedure for taking a sputum sample

Step	Action	Rationale
1 Prepare equipment	Sterile sputum container, gloves, tissues, glass of water, disposable kidney dish, lab. request form, biohazard transport bag, pen to complete documentation	To ensure safe collection of sputum sample and safe storage and transportation.
2 Decontaminate hands	Wash hands or use alcohol rub	To promote infection control and minimize cross infection
3 Explain the procedure to the client		To reassure the client and gain informed consent
4 Ensure the client is in a high sitting position	This will make expectoration a little easier	To minimize discomfort and ensure a good sample is collected. Ensure you support the client in case coughing leads to imbalance
5 Give client the glass of water	Instruct the client to briefly rinse mouth with the water and expel into the kidney dish	This will cleanse the oral cavity and reduce contamination of sample if the client has oral health problems
6 Instruct client to inhale deeply and cough up a sputum and spit a sample into the container	To prevent loss of the sample	To ensure the sample is collected safely, minimizing infection control risk. Offer a tissue to wipe any excess saliva
7 Observe client	In case the process has caused any breathlessness or discomfort	If the client takes inhaler therapy it might be necessary to use this to prevent an asthma attack
8 Collect all equipment for safe disposal	Used equipment should be properly disposed of into normal and clinical waste bags	To support infection control and prevent contamination. Safe disposal of clinical waste is also an important health and safety issue
9 Recording documentation and sending samples	Ensure you are familiar with the standard way of recording a sample being taken and how it is to be transported	The client case notes and appropriate chart should be completed accurately. You may describe the colour, amount, thickness of the sample and any smell that may be present
10 Communicate findings 1	Inform client that the sample has been collected and be prepared to answer any queries they may have	To reassure the client
11 Communicate findings 2	Document that the sample has been taken and sent to the lab. Advise staff that the lab result will be imminent	So that other members of the team are aware that a sample has been sent and to be alert when the result comes back
12 Decontaminate hands	Wash hands or use alcohol rub	To promote infection control and minimize cross infection

Procedure for taking a peak expiratory flow rate reading

See Table 3.14 for a step by step guide to this procedure, with rationales. In the US, the National Heart, Lung and Blood Institute (2007: 59) Expert Panel recommends long-term daily peak flow monitoring for patients who have moderate or severe persistent asthma. They suggest that this

Table 3.14 Procedure for taking a peak expiratory flow rate reading

Step	Action	Rationale
1 Prepare equipment	Peak flow meter, clean once use mouth piece, pen and chart for recording result	To ensure effective monitoring and prompt recording of reading
2 Decontaminate hands	Wash hands or use alcohol rub	To promote infection control and minimize cross infection
3 Explain and demonstrate procedure for the client	Ensure client is paying attention and is clear about what they need to do	To ensure the client knows how to do the procedure and gain consent
4 Ask client to stand and blow into the meter	Ensure client has formed an effective seal around the mouthpiece	To minimize risk of air escaping leading to failed readings
5 Repeat this process for three consecutive readings	Take the best reading as the actual reading	Always observe for poor technique; advise the client that if they feel dizzy they should wait for a few seconds more before next attempt
6 Replace and safely dispose of used equipment	Dispose of single use equipment	To prevent accidental reuse, cross infection
7 Record and document your findings	Ensure you are familiar with the standard way to record and document PEFR readings	The appropriate chart should be completed accurately for comparison with other past, or for future readings
8 Communicate findings 1	Inform client of the outcome and be prepared to answer any queries they may have	To reassure the client
9 Communicate findings 2	Report any abnormalities to the nurse in charge	In case immediate intervention is required or for continuity of care
10 Communicate findings 3	Record findings in the client's case notes	So that other members of the team are aware of them
11 Decontaminate hands again	Wash hands or use alcohol rub	To promote infection control and minimize cross infection

level of monitoring will detect early changes in disease states that require treatment, evaluate responses to changes in therapy and afford a quantitative measure of impairment.

PEFR measurements are usually taken four times per day, both before and after the administration of bronchodilators (out of hospital this is usually twice a day) (Jevon 2007c). When clients are using PEFR this presents practitioners with an opportunity of forming a therapeutic alliance which can increase your health promotion role. Practitioners should also include family and carers in the educational process so that they can be empowered to support their loved one.

Poor technique can lead to inaccurate PEFR readings. You will have to educate the client in proper technique and this will probably entail you role-playing it. Problems with poor PEFR technique include

- Not enveloping the mouth piece correctly so that air escapes
- A coughing or spluttering motion on expiration
- Not taking a deep enough breath
- Not holding the meter correctly so that fingers prevent the arrow moving appropriately

Another aspect of client education will be recording the readings on a chart. Charts are usually supplied with the PEFR meter so you will have to demonstrate the process of recording to clients and their carers.

Urinalysis

Mallett and Dougherty (2000: 424) define urinalysis as 'the testing of the physical characteristics and composition of freshly voided urine'. Urinalysis is a useful, non-invasive test and can be used to obtain a baseline assessment for future comparison, detect abnormalities in urine composition or to monitor the progress of an existing condition. In mental health we also use urinalysis to monitor substance misuse. In my experience this investigation is no longer routinely done on admission. It is more reserved for clients who might present with a 'drug induced' psychosis. However, with the incidence of physical illness rising, it would be appropriate to reintroduce it as a routine observation.

Urine testing can be performed in the clinical area using the standard reagent 'dip sticks' or a urine sample may be sent for more specific pathology testing (see Table 3.15). Urinalysis is a useful screening method for diabetes. Here you will find positive readings for glucose (glycosuria) and ketones (ketonuria). As the body loses weight fat is used as an energy source and this is excreted in urine as ketones. This will also occur in people with eating disorders such as anorexia nervosa.

Citrome *et al.* (2003) found that those taking clozapine were more likely to have glucose screening than those taking other medications. This presents a clear problem when trying to compare typical and atypical medications for prevalence of diabetes. It may also present as an inequality in health care as metabolic risks can occur with all types of antipsychotic medications.

Equipment

For a routine urinalysis test you will need

- Reagent strips
- A secure sample of urine, either in a sample pot or other appropriate container
- A watch with a second hand to time the reagent reaction
- Gloves and an apron in case of splashing

Table 3.15 Different types of urine samples

Type of sample	Use
Specimen for 'dipstick'	A routine urine sample for testing
Catheter specimen of urine (CSU)	A sample that is removed from a catheter. This may require a syringe and needle so be careful of needle stick injury or accidentally perforating the catheter bag
Specimen for cytology	A urine sample sent to a lab for testing, e.g. for a urinary tract infection
Midstream specimen of urine (MSU)	A 'sterile' sample of urine where the person begins to pass urine, stops momentarily and passes a sample into a receptacle
Early morning specimen of urine (EMU)	A sample taken first thing in the morning to ensure 'everything' is tested
24 hour collection	Is used to check kidney function or identify the presence of filtrate such as creatinine. The urine sample should be refrigerated to reduce degradation
Random urine drug screen	If clients are in a drug rehabilitation programme a condition will be staying 'clean'. Random urine screening seeks to detect drug use. This is a normal sample taken at any time, day or night. The client needs to be observed to ensure the sample is their own and not one that is smuggled.

Procedure for urinalysis

This procedure will focus on a midstream sample of urine. First we should ensure the privacy and dignity of the client giving the sample. We should then ensure that they minimize cross infection by providing aids for getting the urine into the receptacle; this might be a clean once use bed pan or urinal bottle. We should also advise the client to wash their hands following this.

Once the sample has been given you should take any supplementary measurements, e.g. in the case of fluid balance accurately record the quantity of urine voided on the chart. Table 3.16 shows the stages in the procedure.

Other aspects of urinalysis

From observation we can tell if there are potential problems with a urine sample. The colour, smell and the presence of floating particles may indicate an infection. However, we must always perform the urinalysis test to get an accurate assessment. You should remember that the colour

Table 3.16 Procedure for urinalysis

Step	Action	Rationale
1 Prepare equipment	Watch with second hand, reagent strips, gloves (possibly an apron also) pen and chart for recording result	To ensure effective monitoring and prompt recording of reading
2 Examine reagent strips	Check that they are not out of date and that they have been stored appropriately.	If out of date or stored inadequately the reagent strip may have reacted to moisture in the air. Do not use as this will give a false reading
3 Take out one reagent strip and replace lid	Do not touch the reagent pads	To minimize biased readings and ensure secure storage for next time
4 Dip reagent strip into the sample	Immerse the reagent strip in the urine sample	To ensure that all reagent pads have been activated
5 Carefully remove the reagent strip	Extract the strip at an angle to allow excess urine to run off safely.	This will prevent excess urine running through the different reagent pads which will affect readings
6 Use your watch to begin timing as reagent pads activate at different times	Ensure readings are taken at the correct intervals	Failure to record at correct intervals will invalidate the readings
7 Record and document your findings	Ensure you are familiar with the standard way of recording urinalysis findings	The appropriate chart should be completed accurately for comparison with other past, or for future readings
8 Communicate findings 1	Inform client of the outcome and be prepared to answer any queries they may have	To reassure the client
9 Communicate findings 2	Report any abnormalities to the nurse in charge	In case immediate intervention is required or for continuity of care
10 Communicate findings 3	Record findings in the client's case notes	So that other members of the team are aware of them
11 Decontaminate hands again	Wash hands or use alcohol rub	To promote infection control and minimize cross infection

of urine may have changed for innocent reasons, e.g. eating beetroot can cause discolouration (BNF 2007). Some antibiotic medication can also cause discolouration, e.g. rifampicin can give urine an orange tinge. Urine normally smells slightly aromatic but diabetes mellitus can give it a fruity smell due to the presence of acetone (Dougherty and Lister 2008).

Abnormalities detected by urinalysis

It is important that you are aware of what each reagent pad on the strip is measuring. Table 3.17 illustrates how urinalysis should be seen within a mental health context and gives both the medical terms that we should be familiar with and possible causes.

Specific gravity in urinalysis

'Specific gravity measures the concentration of urine solutes, which reflects the kidney's capacity to concentrate urine, this capacity is among the first functions lost when renal tubular damage occurs' (Buffington and Turner 2004: 146). It is also referred to as relative density. Using the model of homeostasis, normal specific gravity ranges from 1.010 to 1.025. Specific gravity below 1.010 or above 1.025 may indicate a problem in renal function as the kidneys are not filtering or retaining solutes as they should be.

Table 3.17 Abnormalities found in urinalysis

Substance	Medical term	Possible causes
Glucose	Glycosuria	Diabetes mellitus, total parenteral nutrition (giving IV fluids), sometimes in pregnancy
Bilirubin	Bilirubinuria	Stale urine (if left untested urine will still break down. If stale urine is tested it may mistakenly read as bilirubinuria), liver disease
Ketones	Ketonuria	Diabetic ketoacidosis, vomiting, severe dieting, cachexia (the latter are found in individuals with anorexia)
Low specific gravity		High fluid intake (dipsomania), diabetes insipidus, chronic renal failure, hypokalaemia (low levels of potassium)
High specific gravity		Dehydration (e.g. excessive vomiting), chronic renal failure or cardiac problems
Blood	Haematuria	Menstruation in women, infection, kidney stones, injury to urinary tract, e.g. during catheterization
Low pH (acidic)		High protein diet, diabetic ketoacidosis, starvation (anorexia), hypokalaemia, pyrexia, diarrhoea (laxative abuse)
High pH (alkalinic)		Stale urine, vegetarian diet, urinary tract infection, vomiting (bulemia), metabolic or respiratory acidosis
Protein	Proteinuria	Urinary tract infection, severe hypertension, heart failure, renal failure, pre-eclampsia (practitioners working in mother and baby units should be aware of any history of pre-eclampsia and how this might affect blood pressure)
Urobilinogen	Urobilinogenuria	Liver disease (alcohol misuse)
Nitrite		Infection
Leucocytes	Pyuria	Urinary tract infection

Urine pH

An acidic or alkalinic urine specimen indicates that pH homeostasis is in a state of imbalance. This may suggest a problem with the kidney's ability to maintain a normal pH range.

Urine glucose and ketone tests

Urinalysis can be a useful test in the monitoring of glucose and ketone levels, which are important in screening for type 2 diabetes. However, the standard way of monitoring glucose is through blood glucose testing. The presence of ketones in urine may indicate that the person's own fat reserves are being used as an energy source. Ketones would be evident in cases of anorexia nervosa or diabetic ketoacidosis.

Measuring body mass index

To assess the extent of obesity in our client group we must first know what the standardized measurement of obesity is. Definitions of weight for health purposes are commonly measured on the body mass index (BMI) scale. BMI measurement is recognized globally.

$$BMI = \frac{Weight\ Kg}{Height\ m^2}$$

The BMI score is not gender biased i.e. the same scale and calculation applies to both males and females. The BMI classification and score are illustrated in Table 3.18.

Procedure for measuring BMI

See Table 3.19 for an outline of this procedure in ten steps.

Table 3.18 The International Classification of adult underweight, overweight and obesity according to BMI

Classification	BMI(kg/m²)	
	Principal cut-off points	**Additional cut-off points**
Underweight	<18.50	<18.50
Severe thinness	<16.00	<16.00
Moderate thinness	16.00–16.99	16.00–16.99
Mild thinness	17.00–18.49	17.00–18.49
Normal range	18.50–24.99	18.50–22.99
		23.00–24.99
Overweight	≥25.00	≥25.00
Pre-obese	25.00–29.99	25.00–27.49
		27.50–29.99
Obese	≥30.00	≥30.00
Obese class I	30.00–34–99	30.00–32.49
		32.50–34.99
Obese class II	35.00–39.99	35.00–37.49
		37.50–39.99
Obese class III	≥40.00	≥40.00

Source: WHO (2006)

Table 3.19 Procedure for measuring BMI

Step	Action	Rationale
1 Prepare equipment	Ensure you have functioning scales, a height measurement tool, a BMI calculation chart or a calculator to make the calculation, pen to record reading and documentation	To ensure effective monitoring and prompt recording of reading
2 Explain procedure	Outline your intended actions	To gain consent and reassure the client
3 Ensure privacy	Carry out procedure in a suitable clinical environment	To show respect and preserve dignity
4 Weigh client	Ask client to remove shoes and outer clothes and stand, or sit, on scales. Ensure scales are set to 0	To get an accurate weight (Kgs) measurement
5 Measure client's height	Client can put clothes on again. Ask client to stand erect beside the height measure*	To gain an accurate height (metres) measurement then calculate to m^2
6 Calculate BMI	Use either a visual measure from a chart, or a BMI calculator	To arrive at client's BMI
7 Record and document your findings	Complete appropriate chart	For comparison with other past or future readings
8 Communicate findings 1	Inform client of the outcome and be prepared to answer any queries they may have	To reassure the client
9 Communicate findings 2	Report any abnormalities to the nurse in charge	In case immediate intervention is required or for continuity of care
10 Communicate findings 3	Record findings in the client's case notes	So that other members of the team are aware of them

Note: * If client cannot stand erect then a demispan measurement can be used (Perry 2007). Here height is calculated by measuring one arm outstretched from the base of the middle/ring fingers to the sternal notch using a non-stretch tape measure. The height is calculated for women: height in cm = (1.35 × demispan cm) + 60.1; men: Height in cm = (1.4 × demispan cm) + 57.8 (Perry 2007).

Waist circumference and waist to hip ratio

BMI is not the only measurement of weight. Central (abdominal) obesity is a risk factor for CHD. A simple waist measurement can be a useful risk indicator for obesity. Diabetes UK (2008) suggest that a waist measurement > 94cm (> 37 inches) for white and black men, and > 90cm (> 35 inches) for Asian men, and > 80cm (> 31.5 inches) for white, black and Asian women are risk factors for diabetes. Therefore a target in reducing weight might also include reducing waist size.

Canoy *et al.* (2007: 2941) found that measures of abdominal obesity were more predictive of CHD, stating that reducing waist circumference by 5cm could lower risk by 11 per cent in men and 15 per cent in women. Yusuf *et al.* (2005) determined that waist to hip ratio was more significant in assessing risk of myocardial infarction than BMI. This measurement is a way of determining obesity and may be used in conjunction with the BMI. Hip to waist ratio is calculated by dividing the circumference of the waist by the circumference of the hips.

A healthy waist to hip ratio is

- Women – 0.80 or less
- Men – 0.90
- Anything over 1.0 is considered obese

(Obesity Focused 2008)

Blood glucose measurement

Testing a client's blood for glucose imbalance is an important aspect of caring for a client with diabetes, or for screening for diabetes in your client group. Exposure to blood, albeit in a minuscule quantity, is a risk. Therefore for health and safety it is important that infection control measures are followed regarding disposal of sharps and clinical waste.

Testing blood glucose will give an indication of the client's blood glucose levels. This will enable practitioners to evaluate the success of any lifestyle changes or medication given to regulate blood glucose levels. Diabetes UK (2006) suggest that a normal blood glucose level is

- Fasting (before a meal)   4–6 mmol/l
- Post prandial: (2 hours after food)   less than 10 mmol/l

Blood glucose testing should be done in line with the client's care plan. Depending on the severity this might be done typically before and after meals, e.g. in type 1 diabetes, before and after breakfast, lunch and the evening meal. In type 2 diabetes blood glucose testing may not be required, may be required infrequently, e.g. weekly, or may be required daily. Again this depends on the presence of other risk factors such as having a co-morbid illness.

Normally clients will monitor their own blood glucose levels. When well, the role of the nurse will be to review the client's blood glucose levels in the client's own record. When clients are unwell this may need to be facilitated for them by the practitioner as they may not have the concentration or dexterity to perform it. However, promoting client independence will be a key therapeutic aim in the nursing care plan.

Equipment

Blood glucose is tested using a glucometer. It is important that both practitioner and client are trained in how to use the glucometer correctly. Glucometers usually have a standard disposable lancet and testing strips. It is important that the equipment used is that which is recommended by the manufacturer.

Procedure for a blood glucose reading

Table 3.20 focuses on taking a blood glucose reading using a glucometer. The client should select the finger to be used. It is important that this varies as repeated pricks in the same finger can compromise the skin.

Box 3.9 Case example

Carlos is a 38-year-old male with a history of schizophrenia. He is currently receiving olanzapine 7.5mg twice daily. He smokes 40 cigarettes daily, engages in no physical activity and has a poor diet. He has type 2 diabetes and takes metformin 500mg with meals three times a day. He requires blood glucose monitoring. What do you do?

Table 3.20 Procedure for a blood glucose reading

Step	Action	Rationale
1 Prepare equipment	Select glucometer, disposable lancet, testing strips, gauze, disposable gloves, sharps box, pen, chart for recording result	To ensure effective and safe monitoring and prompt recording of reading
2 Decontaminate hands	Wash hands or use alcohol rub	Both client and staff do this as client's skin will be punctured; this promotes infection control and minimizes cross infection
3 Explain procedure	Outline your intended actions	To reassure the client and gain consent
4 Ensure client is sitting	Make the client is comfortable and prepare them for a small jab	In case the client experiences an unpleasant feeling following the finger prick
5 Check and prepare equipment	Check expiry dates of test strips, check glucometer is working i.e. note battery strength, insert disposable lancet	To ensure a proper reading and that proper test strips are being used
6 Prick the client's finger once	To draw a drop of blood	Wearing the disposable gloves, ensure you are firm but not forceful as only a drop of blood is required. Gently squeeze the site to obtain a bigger droplet if required
7 Cover the test strip pad with some blood	Insert the test strip into the glucometer	Wait the required time for the reading
8 Dispose of used equipment	Use proper sharps box and clinical waste bags	For infection control purposes
9 Record and document your findings	Ensure you are familiar with the standard way of recording this measurement	The appropriate chart should be completed accurately for comparison with other past, or for future readings
10 Communicate findings 1	Inform client of the outcome and be prepared to answer any queries they may have	To reassure the client
11 Communicate findings 2	Report any abnormalities to the nurse in charge	In case immediate intervention is required or for continuity of care
12 Communicate findings 3	Record findings in the client's case notes	So that other members of the team are aware of them
13 Decontaminate hands again	Wash hands or use alcohol rub	To promote infection control and minimize cross infection

Assessment and diagnosis

Carlos has type 2 diabetes which requires monitoring during his respite stay in hospital

Plan

To monitor Carlos's type 2 diabetes as per his current care plan which involves

- Diet and lifestyle factors
- Metformin 500mg three times a day
- Daily blood glucose testing and recording

Implementation

For continuity of care Carlos's current care plan for his type 2 diabetes needs to be monitored during his respite stay:

- Carlos needs to monitor his blood glucose twice daily (1) before breakfast and (2) before going to sleep.
- Promote Carlos's independence by encouraging him to keep to his own testing routine. Carlos should keep his glucometer and other equipment with him. However, testing should occur in the clinical room where used equipment can be safely disposed. Staff should observe Carlos while he is doing the test and recording the reading.
- Carlos should keep a record of his blood glucose readings. Staff should physically check that he is doing this on a regular basis.
- Staff should keep a note of the blood glucose readings in Carlos's case notes.
- Carlos takes metformin 500mg three times daily along with meals. Staff should dispense medication as per NMC (2008) guidelines and ensure that Carlos takes the medication.
- Staff should observe Carlos for both positive and negative side effects of medication.
- Staff should liaise with Carlos's diabetic nurse specialist and share information as appropriate.

Carlos has a reduced calorie diet that he needs to maintain. However, this has proved very challenging and he frequently has problems maintaining it.

- Staff should liaise with the dietician regarding Carlos's diet and explore ways of maintaining it.
- Carlos should be referred to Occupational Therapy for advice on food preparation.
- Carlos should have his blood pressure, pulse, BMI and waist hip ratio recorded and monitored.
- Staff should give Carlos health education and promotion advice.
- Staff should encourage Carlos to be physically active during the day.
- Carlos should be referred to a smoking cessation therapist for advice on how to reduce/stop his smoking.
- Staff should discuss the benefits of stopping smoking with Carlos and introduce him to the idea of nicotine replacement therapy.
- Staff should observe Carlos for both positive and negative side effects of poor diet.
- Ensure night staff are aware of the care plan to reduce Carlos snacking inappropriately at night and to promote continuity of care.
- Regularly monitor the care plan to determine progress.

Evaluate

- Daily evaluation will be conducted at the end of each shift. This will include monitoring baseline observations, blood glucose levels, medication compliance and dietary intake.
- The care plan will be re-evaluated if Carlos experiences any serious complications, e.g. hypoglycaemia or diabetic ketoacidosis.

Blood tests

Box 3.10 **Exercise**	Go to your clinical room and list the different types of blood bottles that are there. Can you match the blood tests with the different bottles?

Testing blood for analysis allows practitioners to

- investigate and diagnose a range of physical conditions
- monitor for presence of infection
- monitor arterial blood gases
- monitor blood glucose levels
- monitor electrolyte levels
- monitor therapeutic ranges for medications

Various blood tests have corresponding 'blood bottles'; vials with different coloured tops which indicate the test. These vials contain different substances, e.g. an anticoagulant to prevent the blood from clotting (if this is a test requirement), vials without an anticoagulant or a serum separator when blood samples need to be put in a centrifuge and separated.

You may not normally take blood unless you have undergone specific phlebotomy training and are deemed competent in undertaking this role. Blood is usually taken by a phlebotomist or a doctor. However, it is important for practitioners to have the background knowledge of what the blood is getting tested for and what this might mean for the client's physical and mental health.

There are a range of different blood tests and here we will examine some that may be described as routine in mental health care. Needless to say, clients may require different tests than those outlined here depending on their individual presentation. This section will be split whereas in reality the tests will probably be components of the full blood count. It should also be remembered that normal ranges may vary slightly from laboratory to laboratory.

Full blood count (FBC)

The FBC is a general analysis of a sample of blood that includes red blood cells, iron levels, white blood cells, platelets, electrolytes and hormones. This test can be very inclusive or specific aspects can be requested, depending on the presenting complaint.

Biochemistry

Biochemistry testing is used to examine electrolyte balance. Having stable electrolyte levels is important for physical health, e.g. monitoring sodium levels is an important factor in cardio-vascular health. When blood is taken and sent to the laboratory the tests that may be requested include those shown in Table 3.22.

Table 3.21 Blood tests and normal values

Blood test	Normal levels
Haemoglobin	14–17.4g/d (male), 12.3–15.3 (female)
Red blood cell count	4.5–5.9 × 10^6/μL (male), 4.5–5.1 × 10^6/μL (female)
Erythrocyte sedimentation rate (ESR)	Adults < 50 years: Male 0–15mm/hr, Female 0–20mm/hr Adult > 50 years 0–30 mm/hr
Platelet count*	150,000–400,000 cells/μL#

Source: Adapted from Malarkey and McMorrow (2005)

* Platelets are also called thrombocytes. Thrombocytopenia is a reduction in platelets which is also a side effect of antipsychotic medications such as clozapine.

\# symbol for microlitre

Table 3.22 Some ranges for bio chemistry blood tests

Electrolyte	Normal range
Sodium	135–145mmol/l
Potassium	3.5–5.5 mmol/l
Creatinine	60–125μmol*/l (men) and 55–110μmol (women)
Calcium	2.15–2.65 mmol/l

* mmol is the symbol for millimole, μmol symbol for micromole

Arterial blood gas

Measurements of blood pH, oxygen and carbon dioxide levels can be obtained from an arterial blood sample. Arterial blood gases (ABGs) perform an important diagnostic and monitoring function for clients with respiratory problems. ABGs assess lung function by illustrating how well the lungs supply oxygen and eliminate carbon dioxide. This helps in diagnosing a physical disorder or monitoring effectiveness of treatment by comparing a range of results to determine how a condition is progressing. Maintaining a stable body pH is also important. An ABG sample may indicate acidosis. If the blood plasma is acidic, respirations will increase in rate and depth to correct this imbalance (see Chapter 6 on respiration).

Causes of abnormal respiratory values (Allibone and Nation 2006):

- Respiratory acidosis or alkalosis
- Inadequate alveolar ventilation
- Excess CO^2 production
- Lung disease e.g. COPD, pneumonia or asthma
- Central nervous system depression due to medication or brain stem injury
- Impaired respiratory muscle function due to chest wall injury or deformity
- Airway obstruction
- Pulmonary oedema
- Cardiac arrest
- Hysteria or anxiety
- Hypoxia

As blood is taken directly from an artery practitioners should have the appropriate competence in this procedure. Your role in this procedure may be as an assistant. Following the procedure, the arm should be elevated and the puncture site compressed until the bleeding stops; this can take up to three minutes (Hastings 2009). It has been reported that patients often experience considerable pain with repeated ABG levels (*Nursing Times* 2002). Practitioners should support clients, allowing them to express feelings and offer reassurance about the necessity and importance of the tests. Educating and preparing the client if a series of ABGs is required may lessen the reluctance for the tests.

Cardiac enzymes

When cell tissue gets damaged it releases enzymes into the blood stream. These act as markers which can be identified in blood tests. In myocarditis, the damaged heart tissue releases its markers, in this case an enzyme called troponin, into the blood stream. This can be identified in a cardiac enzyme blood test. This is an important blood test in clients taking clozapine (see Chapter 8 for adverse drug reactions of medication).

Blood cultures

Testing blood for cultures is a test to determine the presence of infection. This type of test will also indicate the type of antibiotic treatment that may be required to treat the infection.

Hormone levels

Blood tests can also monitor the presence and levels of hormones in circulation, for example, blood glucose levels may indicate problems with insulin tolerance. Other common hormone tests include the thyroid function test which tests for the levels of thyroid stimulating hormone (thyrotropin) in the blood. This test is important as it can serve to differentiate between a poorly functioning thyroid gland and depression (see Table 3.23). Thyroid stimulating hormone normal level for adults is 0.4–4.2 ml/U/L (Malarkey and McMorrow 2009).

Prolactin is another hormone that is usually tested for in response to adverse drug reactions (see Chapter 8). The normal values for prolactin are:

- Females less than 25mcg/L
- Males less than 20mcg/L

Breast enlargement and lactation are natural responses in pregnancy. Therefore pregnancy can elevate the levels of prolactin. In pregnant women the normal range of prolactin is 20–400mcg/L.

Fighting infection

Monitoring white blood cell count is important in determining the presence and severity of infection. In mental health it is also an important measurement for monitoring adverse drug reactions such as neutropenia in anti-psychotics (see Table 3.24).

Table 3.23 Comparing some signs and symptoms of hypothyroidism and depression

Hypothyroidism	Depression
Fatigue	Fatigue
Lack of energy	Lack of energy
Decreased libido	Decreased libido
Low mood	Low mood
Poor concentration	Poor concentration
Poor memory	Poor memory

Table 3.24 White blood cell tests and normal values

Blood test	Normal range
White blood cell count	$4.5–11 \times 10^3/\mu L$ (males),
Differential white blood cell count	
Neutrophils	1,800–7,800 cells µL
Lymphocytes	1,000–4,800 cells µL
Monocytes	0–800 cells µL

Source: Adapted from Malarkey and McMorrow (2005)

Monitoring levels of medication

Some medications require monitoring to ensure that they are within a set therapeutic range. Lithium, which is used to treat bipolar disorder and mania, is probably the most frequent drug test. However, clients with epilepsy also require medication levels checked to monitor therapeutic efficacy and compliance. Some examples of medications and therapeutic ranges include the following (Taylor *et al.* 2005):

- Lithium carbonate: 0.6–1.0 mmol/l
- Carbamazepine: >7 mg/l
- Olanzapine: 20–40 µg/l
- Clozapine: 350–500 µg/l

Summary of key points

- Practitioners are required to have the skills and knowledge to undertake a range of clinical observations.
- Clinical governance issues are very important in ensuring clinical observations are undertaken in a safe and effective manner.
- Clear documentation and communication of results is important for continuity of care.
- Practitioners should undertake regular training updates to ensure their skills base and competency is up to date.

Quick quiz

1 What is the therapeutic range for lithium?
2 What is the normal temperature range for an adult?
3 Define homeostasis.
4 What are the Korotkoff sounds? How many phases are there?
5 List the factors that might affect pulse oximetry readings.

4 Principles of physical health assessment in mental health care

By the end of this chapter you will be able to:

- Explore your role in physical assessment
- Describe the process of physical assessment
- Appreciate the different methods of physical assessment
- Examine equipment essential for physical assessment
- Discuss the importance of privacy, dignity and consent

Box 4.1
Exercise   In which ways can you structure a physical assessment?

Introduction

Earlier chapters have illustrated how our clients have high rates of physical illness that go largely undetected. Indeed a physical condition may go undetected for such long periods of time that it may only become manifest through a critical event, for example, a patient may experience hypoglycaemia which leads to a diagnosis of diabetes. It is important therefore that nurses have the fundamental skills, knowledge and equipment to conduct a thorough physical assessment.

Rushforth *et al.* (1998) suggest that for most nurses, physical assessment is regarded as primarily the recording of vital signs such as temperature, heart rate, respiratory rate and blood pressure. In mental health physical assessment may be constrained, as Rushforth suggests, to taking and recording baseline observations on admission or discharge from hospital. Performing a physical assessment may be a new role requirement and as such it is necessary for practitioners to have appropriate support. Mental health services need to ensure that practitioners are educated and trained to undertake physical assessment with support from an experienced practitioner who might act as a mentor. Clinical supervision should also be considered as part of the support process.

This chapter will examine skills which help facilitate a physical assessment. Mental health nurses will have some skills but these may be 'rusty'. For example research by Nash (2005) found that while practitioners reported having physical care skills, these had been learned as part of their student nurse training and 42 per cent of the sample had been qualified for more than ten years. It is fair to assume that some knowledge and skills may be out of date given advances in evidence based practice. Therefore, training in physical assessment will need to be updated.

Why physical assessment skills?

Why not? We are now familiar with the extent of physical illness and poor health in our client group. Assessment is the basis of good clinical decision making. Physical assessment will give practitioners information on the nature of any physical problem, its severity, its history, the best intervention and best management plan. If no physical assessment is made it leaves the door open for clinical error. You may need to expand your repertoire of physical assessment skills as this can increase the quality of care your clients receive.

Price *et al.* (2000: 292) suggest that 'the role of the nurse undertaking physical assessment is not to make a nursing or a medical diagnosis. It is to facilitate and enhance the care of a patient by collecting information in a standard fashion and communicating it to other members of the clinical team.' This definition should be a benchmark for our practice. The aim of learning these skills is not to become mini-doctors or pseudo 'general' nurses, it is to enhance the skills and scope of our professional practice. Physical assessment need not be too complex, yet it should not be cursory given the extent of hidden morbidity and the presence of highly visible risk factors.

Practical aspects of physical assessment

Practitioners should remember important practical considerations before commencing an assessment. The principles of infection control should be followed according to local policy and procedure. This will include proper hand hygiene and use of disposable equipment where possible, e.g. thermometers. You should always be prepared by having all necessary equipment and paperwork, ensuring observations are recorded in real time as it is easy to forget readings. You should ensure you follow appropriate guidelines for documentation and record keeping (in the UK this will be Nursing and Midwifery Council Guidelines 2007). Being prepared shows professionalism and competence which will reassure the client.

Preserving our clients' dignity and respect is important at all times, but more so during a physical assessment where disrobing may be required. Therefore the environment must be private and conducive to affording dignity and respect. The client might like a family member with them during this and if possible this should be accommodated. You need to consider the use of chaperones when gender or cultural preferences are expressed, for example, Muslim men may want a male nurse to undertake the assessment. When gaining consent, you should give a clear explanation about the assessment in order to reassure the client as to their well-being. This should include any clinical observations that may be required, including any physical specimens.

Physical health is a highly individualized concept so you should adopt a client centred approach to assessment. It is important for the client to feel that their concerns are being taken seriously as they may have been subjected to diagnostic overshadowing on reporting physical symptoms before. For the most part you will be doing 'physicals' on clients you either know or who are 'known' to services. Nevertheless, the practical considerations in Figure 4.1 should be extended to all.

What does physical assessment tell us?

Physical assessment can indicate a number of things about a client's physical health. It will give you information on bodily functions and body systems so that you can

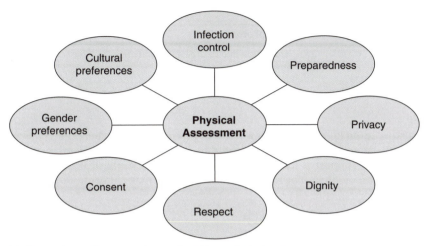

Figure 4.1 Practical considerations when undertaking a physical assessment

- have a baseline measurement for future comparison;
- screen for previously undiagnosed conditions;
- monitor previously diagnosed physical illness;
- determine the response to treatment of a current physical illness;
- monitor the course of a current physical condition;
- prevent increased morbidity by intervening early;
- liaise with the inter-professional team to select the best intervention or treatment.

Physical illness masking and mimicking mental illness

Assessment may also indicate that the presenting mental health problem has an underlying physical cause. Therefore such assessments take on added importance for practitioners working as 'gatekeepers' to mental health services. For example, a nurse working in Accident and Emergency Liaison or Crisis Mental Health Services needs to be aware of physical conditions that may present as acute psychiatric conditions (see Table 4.1). Whatever the purpose of the physical assessment, it is important that practitioners have the appropriate competencies and skills in carrying out a physical assessment.

Core skills in undertaking physical assessment

There is little doubt that the assessment will be based on the medical model of health which focuses on observations being within 'normal' ranges. However, social factors should not be forgotten in this process. While there are different approaches to assessing physical health, the core skills required should be familiar to practitioners. While some of these are technical and manual we should not underestimate the value of our core 'mental health' skills that can be employed in different contexts.

Communication skills

These are the most important mental health nursing skills. During physical assessment you will need to draw on your repertoire of communication and listening skills, especially when

Table 4.1 Physical conditions that may present as acute psychiatric conditions

Physical disorder	Symptoms	Psychiatric disorder
Delirium	Confusion due to urea and electrolyte imbalance	Dementia
Hypothyroidism	Lethargy, lack of energy, tiredness	Depression

discussing intimate and personal aspects of physical health. Therefore verbal and non-verbal skills will be very important when taking a physical history. Clients may also need added psychological support if they are diagnosed as having a physical condition on top of their mental health problem. The following examples of important communication skills are:

Non-verbal communication skills

Show interest by

- having an open body posture, appearing relaxed and confident to dispel unease;
- maintaining eye contact;
- nodding periodically to show attentiveness and understanding;
- keeping an appropriate personal space;
- not frowning or appearing shocked if something intimate is divulged.

Verbal communication skills

We use verbal communication skills in everyday practice. As such there may be nothing new to learn *per se*. However, the use of these verbal skills in a different context may require acclimatization.

Questioning: Open questions are used for global assessment and getting a general picture of the client, e.g. 'How are you feeling today?'

Closed questions are used for more specific assessment e.g. 'Do you drink alcohol?'; 'How many units per week?'

Clarifying: This is used to ensure you have correct information regarding symptoms:

- Have you got the priority correct, e.g. long standing issue or new and acute?
- Paraphrase any unclear statements and try to assign these to a sign or symptom.
- If the assessment is complex summarize at intervals to ensure you have an accurate account.

Listening and responding: You should use attending skills to explore discrepancies in responses. For example, is the client's verbal and non-verbal communication congruent?

Box 4.2 Case example

Nurse: Is there a history of heart disease in your family?
Samuel: (Low tone of voice, no eye contact, hesitant) No.

Samuel's response is guarded and a little incongruent. He may be trying to cope with the stress of a family member having a recent diagnosis of heart disease, a heart attack or death. He may be in denial at present.

Appropriate and timely responses are important during the assessment. This helps to verify information and give more clarity. Responding appropriately may also determine action e.g. is the tachypnoea hyperventilation due to anxiety or a sign of respiratory distress?

Reassuring: Try not to make the client more anxious – they may be unaccustomed to seeing you in a physical health role. It is important to have basic knowledge and skills when it comes to physical assessment. Give explanations of procedures as this will increase the client's confidence in your abilities.

Interpreting verbal cues from the client

In the course of the assessment a past history is taken (see further in this chapter). This will involve asking questions about the client and their family's medical history. This may be stressful for them, especially if they, or a close family member, have had or currently have a medical condition. You should be conscious of any verbal signs. For example:

- Tone: the tone of voice may convey anger or sadness if a serious condition is present.
- Intonation (pitch): this may convey low mood, e.g. if low and monotone, it may indicate problems coping with the challenge of having a physical condition.
- Clarity: the client may offer vague or ambiguous answers regarding symptoms. This should be explored to determine if they are minimizing their illness, or they are articulating it from their own meanings.

Observation

Box 4.3 Exercise	By using observational skills only what type of information about health and illness can you elicit from a patient?

Observation is another core mental health nursing skill. The principle of observation in physical health is the same albeit more technical in recording and reporting baseline observations or signs and symptoms of physical illness. Observation is an important aspect of physical assessment as it can give us important information without asking questions. On first meeting a client there will be a range of information about their physical health that you can elicit from observation. Observation skills are very important for practitioners in situations where clients do not consent to a physical exam. However, when possible observations must be followed up with a structured clinical assessment and not just left to observation alone.

Observation is very important as we can spot signs and symptoms of illness and abnormalities in body systems that can give us important information about a range of aspects of physical health. For example:

- Weight, mobility, personal hygiene – sight
- Body odour, tobacco or alcohol use – smell
- Respiration – hearing

It is important that we use our senses when we 'observe' and do not rely solely on direct question and answering. For example we might smell alcohol on a person's breath, but they may say that they do not drink. This should alert us to this discrepancy which can then be further observed or examined, e.g. checking liver function test on blood results. However, it is important not to assume too much and that appropriate clinical measurements are taken to confirm observations. Table 4.2 illustrates some of the clinical measurements taken during an assessment.

Attitude

A professional attitude is another key assessment skill. You may uncover risk-taking behaviours that run contrary to our health beliefs as health professionals, for example, practising unsafe sex or injecting drug use. A professional attitude will enable you to be non-judgemental so that you can offer appropriate care, support and advice.

Specific techniques

Estes (2002) outlines four key techniques that nurses require in order to perform the physical assessment. Mental health nurses may be unfamiliar with these from a practice perspective but they have most probably seen them employed by a doctor. However, there is no reason for not acquiring these skills and this could be a focus of any training. The four assessment techniques are:

- Inspection: the process of systematic observation using sight and smell;
- Palpation: the use of touch to elicit information such as texture, moisture, temperature, oedema, pulse, shape and size, motion, tenderness or pain;
- Percussion: tapping the body with short, sharp taps to elicit information such as location, size or density;
- Auscultation: using a stethoscope to listen to the sounds produced by the body – breathing, abdominal sounds, heart sounds.

These techniques are then employed in different approaches to physical assessment outlined next.

General approaches to physical assessment

There are three approaches to physical assessment:

- Head to toe approach

Table 4.2 Measurements taken during the course of an assessment

Measurement	Rationale
BMI, girth, waist	Important for diagnosing obesity and monitoring weight which are risk factors for CHD and stroke
Blood pressure, pulse, pulse oximetry	Important for monitoring cardiovascular health, screening for CHD, monitoring medication side effects and oxygen levels in the blood
Temperature	Important for monitoring infections, side effects of medications, e.g. hypothermia
Urinalysis	Important in detecting and monitoring new/existing conditions, e.g. Type 2 diabetes or substance misuse
Respirations, peak flow cough, sputum	Important in monitoring respiratory health, screening for chest infections and measuring lung function
Blood tests	Important to detect, monitor or screen for new/existing conditions e.g. Type 2 diabetes, monitoring medication side effects, e.g. neutropenia

- Body systems approach
- Problem centred approach

The approach to assessment will probably be influenced by a number of considerations (see Table 4.3). However, approaches to assessment are that – approaches. It would not be unusual for a mixture of these to be applied. Approaches are frameworks that serve to help practitioners by giving structure to assessment and a system within which to work. Whichever approach is used it is important that it is structured. It is also important that it is not forgotten in those clients who do not at first consent to it. Most local policies will give a time frame of 72 hours in which this assessment should be completed and it is important that it is followed up within the locally specified timeframes.

Head to toe approach

This is a familiar approach where the nurse takes the person from their head and works down through the body. The assessment focuses on the head, the chest and arms, the abdomen, the groin and legs (see Table 4.4). You will ask questions about

Table 4.3 Factors influencing approaches to physical assessment

Factor	Rationale
The presence of a physical health strategy including the presence of physical assessment documentation	To standardize practice, ensure equity of assessment, prevent ad hoc assessment, provide structure to practice
Standards for physical assessment	To benchmark best practice, provide data for evidence based practice
The role of the doctor in physical assessment	To prevent role or task duplication with the MHN
The mental health status of the client in relation to consent	What to do if consent is not given – see physical assessment of the non-consenting patient later in this chapter (p. 75)
The presence of a pre-existing physical condition	Get collateral information regarding diagnosis and treatment, ensure continuity of care
The presence of a medical condition as the result of a critical incident, e.g. neck injury following attempted asphyxiation	Physical assessment will include observation of all risk factors and safety of both mental and physical health

Table 4.4 Illustrating the head to toe approach in physical assessment

	Factor	Observation	Clinical measurement
General health survey	What is openly visible and observable, not necessarily measurable. This is a non-invasive assessment		
	General appearance	Unkempt, dishevelled Hair – infestation Skin – general condition, colour, tone. Cyanosis, pallor, flushing. Presence of disorders such as eczema or psoriasis, rashes, sores, ulcers, bruising, cuts Nails – broken, split, breaking	Mostly through observation Inspection may be required also (*Continued Overleaf*)

Table 4.4 Continued

	Factor	Observation	Clinical measurement
	Performance of daily activities	Self-care, personal hygiene, body odour, appropriate dress	
	Smoking status	Nicotine stained fingers or hair, smell of tobacco on skin/clothes	Inspection
	Alcohol/drug use	Smell of alcohol, possession of alcohol. Evidence of jaundice – skin yellowing, yellowing of eye sclera	Inspection
		Possession of drugs, needle marks	
	Weight	Appears over or under weight, malnourished	BMI, Malnutrition Universal Screening Tool (MUST) Assessment, girth measurement
	Behaviour	Agitated, fatigued	Self report, direct observation
	Past medical history	Past surgical history History of immunizations	Case notes or self report, inspection
	Signs of obvious injury	Presence of cuts, abrasions, bruises (old or new), visible bandaging or plastering. Presence of sutures – nylon or paper	Self report if not visible, inspection
	Allergies	Signs of allergic reaction – itching, sneezing, allergies to any medications	Self report if not visible, direct observation
Head	Sensory	Sight – wears glasses or contact lenses, eye pain, red or swollen eyes, presence of discharge, self reported visibility problems, blurred vision, nystagmus Hearing – has a hearing aid, complains of earache or ringing in the ears or deafness, discharge from the ear; on examination swollen inner ear	Observation and inspection Observation and self report
	Oral health	Has dentures, state of teeth – broken, missing, halitosis, tongue abrasions/ coated, mouth ulcers, gum problems	Observation, inspection and self report
	Head / neurological	Headache – duration, location, frequency, pain relief, past history of head injury, family history of stroke, experiences migraine, epilepsy, problems with gait, concentration memory	Self report Glasgow Coma Scale, **P**upils **E**qual **R**ound a**n**d **R**eactive to **L**ight (PEARRL)
Neck and chest	Trachea/oesophagus	History of sore throats, swallowing problems, swollen glands, thyroid associated problems, tracheal trauma	Self report, observation, inspection, palpation

	Chest and lungs	Shortness of breath, pain on respiration, laboured breathing, wheeze, cough (dry or productive), past history of respiratory illness – chest infections, COPD, current asthma, smoking history, use of accessory muscles, finger clubbing	Inspection, palpation respiratory rate, pulse oximetry, arterial blood gas, peak flow, spirometry, chest x-ray, sputum sample for pathology
	Chest and heart	Chest pain, hypertension, tachycardia/bradycardia, oedema in hands/ankles	Blood pressure, pulse, electrocardiogram
Abdomen	Gastro-intestinal	Alimentary problems, digestion, elimination	Self-report
		Pain, nausea, vomiting, decreased or increased appetite, gastric reflux, heartburn, abdominal cramping	Inspection, palpation auscultation, self report
		Incontinence – faecal, urinary, constipation	Self report or direct observation
		Pain, frequency, urgency, retention or difficulty in micturation, colour/smell of urine, presence of blood in urine or stool	Urinalysis, urine or stool sample for pathology
Sexual	Women	Menstruation problems, breast lumps	Inspection, palpation pregnancy test, prolactin blood levels, breast screening, mammography, cervical smear for screening
	Men	Impotence, anorgasmia (failure to ejaculate), testicular lumps	Inspection, palpation prolactin blood levels, testicular screening
	Both	Sexual activity and use of contraception, visible discharges, odours, presence/history of rashes indicative of a sexually transmitted disease (STD)	Inspection, self report, blood screening for possible STD, referral for pre-test HIV counselling if appropriate
Musculo-skeletal	Mobility	Steadiness of gait, use of walking aid	Self report, direct observation
	Limbs	Wrist or ankle swelling (oedema), numbness, sensations, peripheral coldness, cyanosis	Inspection, palpation blood tests, e.g. renal function test, sodium or potassium levels, self report, direct observation, touch

- normal and usual functioning;
- changes in functioning;
- pain or discomfort.

Following the assessment laboratory or pathology tests may be required and it is important to gain informed consent if bloods are to be taken. For example, a client may want to know if they have an STD so a blood sample can be taken and sent to the lab. However, if a client wants to know their HIV status, this normally requires pre and post test counselling and you should consult your local policy regarding HIV screening.

Box 4.4   What is the recommended weekly alcohol unit intake for men and women?
Exercise

Body systems approach

This approach requires examination of each body system to determine level of functioning. In nursing journals there are usually skills sections that explore these systems, for example, e.g. in the UK the *Nursing Times* ran a series on 'systems of life' and from this you can structure the assessment (see table 4.5). However, many of the tests of function will be invasive, e.g. blood will be required to assess circulatory and endocrine systems. While not as invasive as taking bloods, blood pressure and temperature will require bodily contact with the client. A body systems approach will include the elements shown in Table 4.5.

Table 4.5 Illustrating the body systems approach to physical assessment

Body system	Example of investigation
General health survey (see above)	
Sensory	eyesight test, hearing test, pain scale
Cardiovascular system	blood pressure, pulse, pulse oximetry, ECG
Blood	range of blood tests, e.g. full blood count, fasting blood glucose, white cell count, cholesterol level
Respiratory system	number of respirations, spirometry, peak flow, blood gases
Gastrointestinal system	questions on bowel movement, listening for bowel sounds, testing stool samples, past operations, e.g. appendicectomy, gall stones
Igumentory systems	inspecting the skin for visible signs of injury or lack of integrity, skin colour, temperature, Waterlow Scale to assess risk of ulcers
Genitourinary system	urinalysis, specimens for pathology, e.g. STDs
Nervous system	levels of consciousness (Glasgow Coma Scale), headaches, irritability, poor concentration
Endocrine system	range of blood tests, e.g. thyroid function
Musculoskeletal	gait, presence of musculoskeletal disorders – arthritis
Other	allergies

Problem centred approach

Another approach to assessment is a problem centred one. Here you will ask the client about the presence of illness, pain or discomfort. If something is identified then specific observations and investigations are then structured around the presenting complaint. Following this you will then take routine observations, general survey and health history that were not part of the problem based assessment (see Figure 4.2).

If there is a presenting complaint encourage the client to be brief and succinct in details. Questions that may act as prompts during the problem based assessment include:

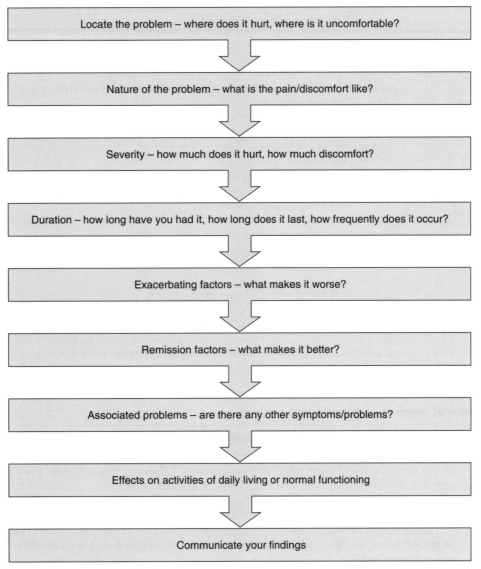

Locate the problem – where does it hurt, where is it uncomfortable?

Nature of the problem – what is the pain/discomfort like?

Severity – how much does it hurt, how much discomfort?

Duration – how long have you had it, how long does it last, how frequently does it occur?

Exacerbating factors – what makes it worse?

Remission factors – what makes it better?

Associated problems – are there any other symptoms/problems?

Effects on activities of daily living or normal functioning

Communicate your findings

Figure 4.2 Structure of a problem based assessment

Timing: Onset – sudden or slow?
           When did it first happen?
           How long has it been going on for?
Pattern: How long does it last for?
           When is it most problematic?
           How often does it happen?
           If pain – is it sharp and stabbing or dull and pulsating?
Severity: Does it stop you doing anything?
           What increases the discomfort?
           What decreases it?
           Have you seen a doctor about it?
           Are you currently getting treatment?

Box 4.5 Case example

Nurse: Hello John, you are due for a physical check, can I do it now?
John: Yes, that's fine.
Nurse: How have you been in general?
John: OK, but I have a bad cough at times.
Nurse: Tell me about the cough, is it a productive cough, I mean do you cough up anything?
John: Yes, sometimes I have some phlegm.
Nurse: You say sometimes, how often is this on a scale of 1 to 10. 1 being all the time and 10 being almost never.
John: I would give it a seven.
Nurse: You say you cough up phlegm, does it have a colour?
John: Yes it is usually greenish.

Given the prevalence of increased morbidity in our clients, there is a likelihood of more than one presenting complaint, for example, cough, chest pain, difficulty in breathing (see Box 4.5). Therefore the initial part of the assessment should be concise. Here practitioners need to decide if the complaints are of a medical emergency – for example, someone is cyanosed and clutching at their chest, or they are anxious and hyperventilating. Problems should therefore be listed in order of severity to prioritize needs safely and give further structure to the assessment.

Physical assessment and history taking

History taking is another core component of physical assessment that practitioners need to become familiar with. History taking is the systematic assessment of key physical health events or risk factors that the client may have experienced. Exploring family history is an important aspect of this in respect to diabetes and coronary problems.

When taking a health history it is important that both open and closed questions are used. The first few questions should be open ended to get the client talking about their general health and lifestyle, how they have been feeling, if they have any concerns or are currently feeling any physical discomfort. From this you can then hone in on any concerns that they have by asking more closed questions.

When taking a health history you should be aware of:

- birth complications and normal developmental milestones, e.g. puberty;
- any pre-existing physical conditions;
- current or past treatment history (as appropriate);
- history of surgery or other significant hospital admissions for a physical problem;
- history of vaccinations and immunizations;
- history of screening, e.g. cervical smear results;
- allergies – in general, e.g. hay fever, more specific adverse drug reactions and drug allergies;
- substance use – alcohol, tobacco, illicit substances.

Taking a family history

Family history is another aspect of physical assessment as conditions such as diabetes and CHD run in families. Although the client may not have a physical condition, if it is part of the family history then it is an important risk factor that needs documenting.

Here you should elicit

- current health status of close family – parents and siblings;
- current physical conditions and treatments;
- past physical conditions and treatments;
- the cause of death if family members have died.

Linking the structure and process during the physical assessment

As stated previously structure is integral to a successful physical assessment. Practitioners must blend the approach to assessment with a process of eliciting information. Figure 4.3 is a

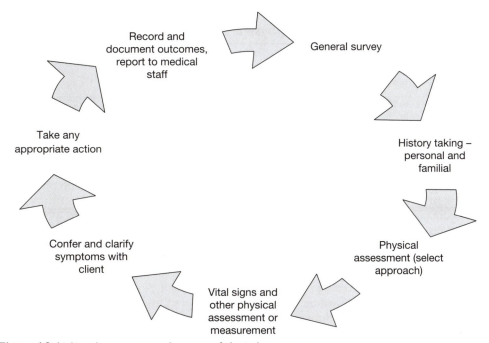

Figure 4.3 Linking the structure and process of physical assessment

representation of this. There is no hard and fast rule to this and as you become more confident and skilled you will undoubtedly find your own style. However, it remains that assessment must be holistic, all observations taken and recorded accurately and communicated to the team and the client. These must be appropriate with timely follow up and onward referral if something is detected.

Essential equipment for a physical assessment

It is important that appropriate equipment is available in order to ensure accurate clinical observations are recorded. It is also important to ensure that any digital equipment used is regularly serviced under the manufacturer's guidelines. Other equipment might be sterile and single use so check expiry dates. The following list illustrates equipment required for a physical assessment:

- Physical assessment checklist
- Associated charts e.g. TPR
- Pen and pocket torch
- Watch with a second hand
- Stethoscope
- Sphygmomanometer
- Thermometer
- Scales, height and waist tape measure
- Urinalysis equipment

Garden (2005) outlines equipment required for a medical assessment and includes some of the above plus an auroscope, alcometer, Snellen chart, tendon hammer and tuning fork (256 Hz).

Issues concerning consent and physical assessment

Box 4.6 Exercise	John is formally admitted to your ward and is detained there for legal reasons. He is agitated and does not want to be there. Suffice to say he does not consent to a physical assessment. From your observations you notice that John is sweaty and a little agitated. You also notice a sweet pear drop odour on his breath. He is not consenting to an assessment. What do you do?

It is important that you gain client consent when undertaking an assessment. At times consent might be implied, for example, when doing physical 'obs' you approach a client with a sphygmomanometer and they begin to roll up their sleeve. It is not only courteous for you to begin by asking if you can perform the observation, it provides you with an opportunity to inquire about the client's health in general. I have witnessed qualified and unqualified nurses presuming consent, strapping on a cuff, pumping it up, recording the reading and leaving without any interaction whatsoever, or any regard for dignity or privacy.

There is no need to overcomplicate the issue of consent. Normally clients will consent to the physical assessment. However, you should be aware of socio-cultural factors that may impact on consent, for example, culture or gender issues concerning male/female nurses and male/female clients. Clients have the right to ask that a nurse of their own gender conduct the physical assessment. For nurses there may still be professional taboos around male nurses undertaking physical assessments on female clients. Ironically this may not be an issue for female nurses and male clients.

At times clients may not consent to a physical assessment. This will probably be at an acute phase of their illness, e.g. following relapse. The client may have been brought to hospital involuntarily and therefore be upset and angry and manifest this by refusal to engage with the admission process (see Box 4.6). In an agitated state, the last thing they need is to be further 'annoyed' by invasive testing, never mind that agitation will probably not give reliable readings for pulse or blood pressure.

Usually physical care protocols will have built in 'clauses' for such situations, e.g. the assessment should happen within 48 or 72 hours of admission. This gives some time for the client to 'settle'. However, it may be easy to miss the assessment altogether if no one goes back to recheck.

Box 4.7 **Exercise**	What systems can be employed to ensure physical assessments are completed?

Physical assessment of a non-consenting client

A client may not consent to a physical exam so invasive measurements such as blood pressure and pulse may not be possible. However, you can still use your observational skills to survey, report and document a 'crude', or simple, assessment until such time as consent is given for a full one (see Table 4.6). The purpose of doing a simple assessment is to notice anything that may require urgent treatment as not to do so may endanger the health and well-being of the client.

Documentation and record keeping

Documenting and recording the physical assessment is very important. You should accurately and clearly document

* what has occurred
* when it has occurred

Table 4.6 A 'simple' physical assessment format for a non-consenting patient

Assessment	Clinical observation
General health survey	General appearance, personal hygiene – body odour, smoking status – tobacco odour, nicotine stains on fingers or hair, smell of alcohol on breath
Sensory	Wears glasses, has a hearing aid
Cardiovascular system	Pallor, cyanosis
Respiratory system	Number of respirations, wheezing, breathlessness, cough
Igumentory systems	Visible signs of injury, bruising (old and recent), dryness, eczema, sweating, skin colour
Nervous system	Level of consciousness, irritability
Endocrine system	Fruity smell on breath
Musculoskeletal	Gait, presence of musculoskeletal disorders – arthritis
Other	Allergies

- what else needs to be done
- by whom
- by when.

It is likely that standardized documentation will be in use so compliance with completing this is important. All clinical measurements should be given, even if they fall into 'normal' ranges or if no problems are noted. For example, it may be assumed that a blank entry means 'no problem noted' but it may also indicate that this part of the assessment has been omitted. Where consent has not been given this should also be documented.

Following the documentation process the outcomes of the assessment will need to be communicated appropriately to:

- the relevant person in charge of the shift (if in a hospital setting);
- the medical staff – including the consultant and any junior doctor;
- the GP (if in the community, residential care or hostel setting);
- the primary nurse or key worker (if they have not been involved);
- other members of the inter-professional team for care planning purposes, e.g. occupational therapist or dietician;
- the client and their family/carer as appropriate.

Inter-professional communication is important for continuity of care especially if further investigations are required. Written communication should be documented under any professional codes of conduct and for nurses this would be the UK Nursing and Midwifery Council (NMC) Code of Standards of Conduct (NMC 2007).

Barriers to using physical assessment skills

Brown *et al.* (1987), suggest that a lack of confidence among some nurses is a barrier to using skills. This highlights the need for robust educational programmes, skills rehearsal and supervised practice, as well as a sound evidence base to underpin practice developments.

There is no general agreement on what should be undertaken as part of a physical assessment nor to aspects of frequency of assessment, e.g. whether it is six monthly or yearly. This general disagreement means that there is no standardized physical assessment tool for use in mental health services, so each constructs their own. Without standardization there may be variations in practice regarding the quality of physical assessment, which might affect the quality of care the client receives. However, useful guidelines for monitoring physical assessment are contained in the UK National Institute for Health and Clinical Excellence (NICE) clinical guideline for bipolar disorder (NICE 2006a):

- People with bipolar disorder should have an annual physical health review, normally in primary care, to ensure that the following are assessed each year:
- lipid levels, including cholesterol in all patients over 40 even if there is no other indication of risk
- plasma glucose levels
- weight
- smoking status and alcohol use
- blood pressure

There is a clear need to have standardized assessment frameworks for initial and annual assessment. This should include the areas shown in Table 4.7 but it is not exclusive.

Table 4.7 An example of an annual health check

Areas for Annual Health Check	
General HE & HP advice Promotion of a healthy lifestyle	Sexual health
New physical conditions	Oral hygiene
Cardio assessment Blood pressure and pulse	Physical activity Exercise
Respiratory assessment Respiratory rate Smoking and smoking cessation	Allergies
Diet and nutrition BMI Cholesterol	Immunization – flu and/or pneumococcal, TB
Endocrine assessment Urinalysis Blood glucose	Screening Self screening of testes or breasts Hepatitis status
Alcohol and/or drug use	

Conclusion

The key to good physical assessment is structure. This chapter has outlined three approaches that can be used as frameworks to structure physical assessment. Within this observation and communication skills are utilized as well as safe and competent clinical skills for clinical measurement. Furthermore, nurses should have basic knowledge of signs and symptoms indicative of physical illness. We have seen that observation is a key skill as a lot of useful information (signs) can be collected, e.g. jaundice or cyanosis. Although nurses may have sound skills for undertaking the 'classic' observations – pulse, blood pressure and temperature – further examination skills should be learned to enhance both competence and confidence in physical assessment. Finally, nurses need to be supported in this role and have appropriate supervision or mentoring.

Summary of key points

- Physical assessment must be structured and physical assessment schedules fully completed.
- Practitioners must be aware of physical illnesses which might present as mental illness.
- Practitioners must have the necessary tools for conducting a physical assessment.
- A structured history is an important part of physical assessment.
- Practitioners must have appropriate physical examination skills, e.g. inspection, palpation, percussion and auscultation.

Quick quiz

1 What practical considerations should the MHN consider in physical assessment?

2 In which ways might the role of the MHN and doctor be duplicated in physical assessment?

3 What will a structured physical assessment tell the MHN about the state of the client's physical health?

4 What aspects of family history are important considerations for the client's physical health?

5 List your own training and education needs in relation to physical assessment.

5 Physical assessment: assessing cardiovascular health

By the end of this chapter you will have:

- Explored the epidemiology of cardio vascular illness in our clients
- Examined risk factors for coronary heart disease in clients
- Outlined the structure and function of the heart
- Described the cardiac cycle and the electrical conduction system of the heart
- Explored the importance of cardiovascular function in clients
- Considered ways of reducing the risks of developing cardiovascular disease

Box 5.1
Exercise
What are the risk factors for cardiovascular illness in your client group?

Introduction

Cardiovascular disease encompasses coronary heart disease (CHD), stroke and peripheral vascular disease (Daniels 2002). CHD is a great threat to public health causing governments worldwide to set targets for reducing the mortality and morbidity rates from it. The World Health Organization (WHO) states that CHD is now the leading cause of death worldwide causing 48.6 per cent of deaths in 2000 (Aboderin *et al.* 2002).

In the UK, CHD accounts for the following (DH 2000b):

- More than 110,000 deaths in England every year.
- More than 1.4 million people suffer from angina.
- Around 300,000 have heart attacks every year.

However, within the picture of CHD in the general population is the story of CHD in our client group. Research statistics illustrate just how big a problem it is:

- People with severe mental illness are over twice as likely to die from cardiovascular disease than someone from the general population (Harris and Barraclough 1998).
- 31 per cent of people with schizophrenia and CHD are diagnosed under 55, compared with 18 per cent of others with CHD.
- 22 per cent of people with CHD who have schizophrenia have died, compared with 8 per cent of people with no serious mental health problems.

(Disability Rights Commission 2006)

Risk factors affecting cardiovascular function

Risk factors for cardiovascular disorders include lifestyle factors such as poor diet, lack of exercise, smoking and alcohol consumption, which can contribute to obesity, high cholesterol, hypertension and diabetes. These factors are present in the general population and our client group. However, our clients are more exposed to these risk factors. In a study of 101 people with severe mental illness living in the community Kendrick (1996) found

- 26 were obese (body mass index greater than 30);
- 53 were current smokers; and
- 11 were hypertensive.

Our clients may also experience poor cardiovascular health due to adverse drug reactions. However, it will most likely be due to a combination of these factors. Other reasons for increased prevalence are also important. Our clients are socially excluded and have poor access to health services and may only present following a critical event, e.g. a heart attack. Signs and symptoms may be recognized but diagnostic overshadowing may interpret tachycardia and hypertension as 'normal' stress reactions to coping with mental illness rather than a 'credible' heart condition.

Whatever the reason, cardiovascular conditions are becoming a common feature of mental health nursing care. Practitioners require safe and competent clinical skills for the assessment, treatment, management and evaluation of care in this area (see Table 5.1).

Does caffeine affect blood pressure?

Caffeine is a stimulant found in coffee, tea, chocolate, cola and energy drinks (NDARC no date). Caffeine in amounts roughly equivalent to several cups of coffee can significantly elevate resting blood pressure in people who don't usually drink it (Lane 1983). Frequent coffee drinkers may develop a tolerance to the increased blood pressure resulting from caffeine intake but Lane suggests that if the same range of blood pressure elevation in people who don't drink coffee registered in those with heart problems there could be complications.

Caffeine intake in clients may not be a problem. However, if caffeine intake is excessive (De Freitas and Schwatrz 1979 found patients drinking 9–10 cups of coffee per day) and linked to other coronary risk factors for high blood pressure then a cumulative effect may increase the risk of coronary problems. For example, a client experiencing **stress** may have a **coffee** to relax. This might include **two or three spoonfuls of sugar**. They may also **smoke** with their coffee. Add to this risk factors such as **lack of exercise, obesity and psychotropic medications**. Now multiply this by a conservative **four cups of coffee per day** for one week and the potential risk may become clear.

Table 5.1 Factors affecting cardiac function

Demographic factors	Age, gender, culture, social class
Lifestyle factors	Sedentary lifestyle (lack of exercise), smoking, high fat diet, high alcohol intake, substance misuse
Psychological factors	Stress and depression
Physiological factors	Atherosclerosis, hypertension and diabetes
Medication	Psychotropic medication – atypical and typical anti-psychotics, tricyclic antidepressants, poly-pharmacy and rapid tranquillization Heart medications – these alter heart function

Ethnicity and hypertension

People from African Caribbean populations have a higher prevalence of hypertension than their white counterparts (BHF 2007a). People from this group are over-represented in compulsory psychiatric admissions (Mental Health Act Commission 1999) and are more likely to be treated with anti-psychotic medications (Lloyd and Moodley 1992). Therefore they should be treated as a high risk group for cardiovascular screening.

Anatomy and physiology of the cardiovascular system

The cardiovascular system consists of the blood, the heart and a closed system of blood vessels (Meurier 2005). The cardiovascular system is responsible for

- blood flow through the body;
- relaying oxygenated blood to tissues and organs;
- returning deoxygenated blood to the lungs;
- carrying nutrients to cells;
- taking waste products for elimination;
- carrying messages to organs and cells via hormones;
- carrying medications to different sites in the body.

Structure of the heart

The heart has four different chambers – the left and right atria which are in the upper portion and the left and right ventricles in the lower portion (see Figure 5.1). Each of the chambers is separated by four different valves that act to prevent the backflow of blood.

There are three different layers of heart tissue:

- The pericardium, the outermost layer, has two components: the fibrous pericardium acts to prevent the heart from over extending and keeps it in place in the chest cavity and the

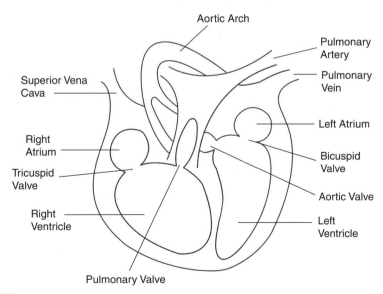

Figure 5.1 The heart chambers and major vessels

serous pericardium serves to lubricate the heart preventing friction during systole and diastole.

- The myocardium, the middle layer of the heart tissue, contains cardiac muscle fibres that allow the heart to contract during beating.
- The endocardium, the inner most layer of smooth membrane, permits the easy flow of blood through the heart.

The heart requires its own blood supply and the myocardium receives this from the right and left coronary arteries. Most of the blood comes during diastole. Deoxygenated blood leaves the heart via the cardiac veins and returns to the right atrium where it is taken to the lungs.

How the heart works

The heart is a muscle that pumps deoxygenated blood to the lungs where it is oxygenated, returned to the heart and pumped around the body. Heart function is controlled and regulated by a series of electric impulses which cause two types of contractions and relaxations – the systole and diastole. We use these for blood pressure measurement. The systolic and diastolic pressures make up the cardiac cycle.

Blood flow through the heart

Venous (deoxygenated) blood returns from the body to the right atrium via the superior and inferior vena cava. It passes from the right atrium through the right atrio-ventricular valve into the right ventricle. This deoxygenated blood is then pumped into the pulmonary artery through the pulmonary valve, which closes to prevent backflow into the right ventricle. From here it goes to the lungs where gaseous exchange occurs – carbon dioxide out and oxygen in. The oxygenated blood is then sent to the left atrium. Here it passes through the mitral valve into the left ventricle. The blood is then forced into the aorta through the aortic valve. The aortic valve closes and prevents back flow of blood into the left ventricle. The blood is then pumped around the body.

The cardiac conduction system

There is more to the heart than the pumping mechanism. The heart also requires a 'shock' to make it beat so it has an electrical system referred to as the cardiac conduction system (see Figure 5.2). This allows the heart to expand and contract at a regular pace. This system is comprised of:

- the sinoatrial node (SA node);
- the atrioventricular node (AV node);
- the atrioventricular bundle (AV bundle or bundle of His) which divides into right and left bundles.

Fibres in the SA node are located in the right atrium wall and act as the heart's pacemaker. During a heartbeat an electrical signal is set off in the SA node which causes the atria to contract, pushing blood into the ventricles. The signal then travels to the AV node and through the AV bundle (or bundle of His) down the left and right bundle branches and disperses around the Purkinje fibres. This causes the ventricles to contract and push blood into the major blood vessels. Oxygenated blood goes into the aorta to be carried around the body and deoxygenated blood goes into the pulmonary artery which goes to the lungs. Here blood is re-oxygenated and returned to the heart and the cycle begins again.

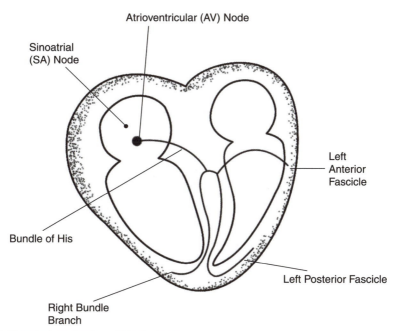

Figure 5.2 Electrical conduction within the heart

Cardiac repolarization

Cardiac conduction relies on a process of depolarization and repolarization. When the heart is about to pump the electrical activity increases causing the ventricles to depolarize and contract (systole) pumping blood out of the heart. The heart muscle then repolarizes and relaxes (diastole) allowing blood to enter for the next heart beat.

Cardiac electrical activity: PQRST waves

The electrical activity of the heart is represented in an electrocardiogram (ECG) reading (see Figure 5.3). The different electrical phases of the ECG are:

- The P wave is associated with atrial activation.
- The QRS wave is associated with ventricular activation.
- ST is the relaxation of the ventricles.
- The T wave signifies the recovery of the ventricular muscle.

(Webster and Thompson 2006)

The QT interval is a measure of the heart's electrical conduction. When these waves occur in harmony we have a normal cardiac cycle. When these waves are disharmonious – either too quick (tachycardia) or too slow (bradycardia) – then we have an abnormal cardiac cycle. This is referred to as cardiac arrhythmia. O'Brien and Oyebode (2003) report that normal QT values are not universally established as factors such as gender (longer in females), time of day, diet, heart rate and selection of ECG leads can cause differences. However, Marder *et al.* (2004) state that the average QT interval is 400msec in healthy adults and a QT interval of 500msec or greater is considered a risk factor for sudden death.

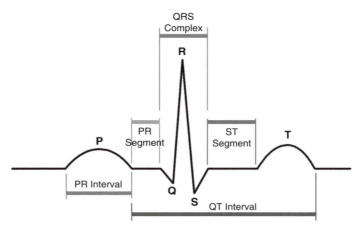

Figure 5.3 Normal ECG reading

The cardiac cycle

The cardiac cycle is the product of the pumping mechanism and the cardiac conduction system. Each set of completed and coordinated cardiac activity is referred to a cardiac cycle. The cardiac cycle consists of

- atrial systole – contraction of the atria;
- ventricular systole – contraction of the ventricles;
- complete cardiac diastole – relaxation of atria and ventricles.

Each cardiac cycle has a cardiac output which is the volume of blood ejected per minute from the left ventricle (Meurier 2005) while the stroke volume is the amount of blood pumped out by a ventricle with each contraction (Dougherty and Lister 2008). Blood pressure and pulse are two ways of measuring cardiac output.

The significance of this for MHNs

Our clients have many risk factors for cardiovascular illness which is often referred to as a silent killer. Although we may have covered basic anatomy and physiology during our student nurse training, this knowledge may lie unused in our memory: 'Since we work in mental health why do we need to know about anatomy and physiology?' However, knowledge of cardiovascular function is important for monitoring our client's physical health. Furthermore, qualified nurses will be mentoring students who will have this knowledge fresh in their minds and may ask questions that might leave us struggling for answers. This will not give learners a good impression.

Box 5.2   List the factors that affect cardiac functioning.
Exercise

Pathophysiology of CHD

When a healthy heart is put under stress the pumping mechanism and the conduction system will work in harmony, responding in a coordinated way to increased heart rate.

When a problem occurs, heart function becomes uncoordinated where the pumping mechanism becomes too fast or too slow and the conduction system emits irregular electrical impulses.

Unhealthy lifestyle factors increase the risk of CHD which is a leading cause of cardiovascular problems. The main cause of CHD is atherosclerosis. Atherosclerosis is a common arterial disorder where plaques of cholesterol, lipids and cell debris form in the inner arterial wall (Anderson and Anderson 1995). This fatty material is called atheroma. Because the atheroma is a foreign body white blood cells attack it. These white cells are called macrophages and these envelop the foreign bodies and form foam cells (Samar 1999).

As blood flow becomes impeded the heart is still pumping the same volume of blood through a reduced arterial space. At rest this may not be a problem. However, as heart rate increases, for example, due to exertion or anxiety this will cause discomfort or pain depending on the severity of the blockage. A small blockage may cause minor discomfort because blood can still flow through. However, a large blockage of 50 per cent or more causes a decrease in blood flow and the heart compensates for this by beating more quickly. This can lead to angina, or, in the event of total blockage of the artery, myocardial infarction.

Not all chest pain will indicate a coronary condition. Tough (2004) outlines various causes of chest pain

- Cardiovascular: myocardial infarction, acute coronary syndrome, angina, pericarditis, aortic aneurysm;
- Pulmonary: pleurisy, pulmonary embolism, pneumothorax, pneumonia;
- Musculoskeletal: costochondritis (inflammation of the rib at point of attachment to the sternum), trauma;
- Gastro-intestinal: reflux, ulcers, gallstones, pancreatitis;
- Psychological: anxiety.

These are important differential diagnoses. Understanding these will enable you to focus your assessment questions, provide appropriate client care and communicate any findings to the inter-professional team.

Disorders of the cardiovascular system

There are three main complications associated with atherosclerosis

- Tissue ischaemia: the heart requires a continuous supply of blood and oxygen. Atherosclerosis causes CHD which leads to decreased perfusion of the myocardium due to blockage of the coronary arteries. When oxygen supply is insufficient to meet the metabolic demands of the affected area, myocardial ischaemia occurs (Hand 2001). Reduced blood and oxygen

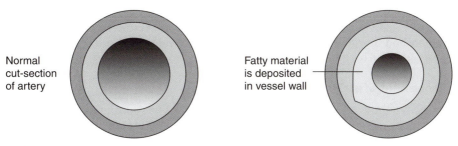

Normal cut-section of artery

Fatty material is deposited in vessel wall

Figure 5.4

supply to the heart muscle causes parts of it to die. Transient ischaemic attacks (TIAs) can occur with decreased blood supply leading to palpitations. This cell death weakens the heart and the more severe this becomes the more heart function deteriorates.

- Myocardial infarction: infarction is the term given to tissue death because of interrupted blood supply (Waugh and Grant 2006). Acute myocardial infarction is the sudden occlusion of a coronary artery leading to myocardial cell death and heart failure (Resuscitation Council UK 2004). However, other complications may occur. If the blockage breaks down a blood clot may enter the circulatory system. This embolism can lodge in smaller arteries causing problems to the periphery or in serious cases pulmonary embolism, a clot to the lungs, or stroke.

- Aneurysm: when arterial walls are damaged they are repaired by fibrous cells, which are not as flexible as cardiac cells. This makes the artery vulnerable to tearing or protrusion. An aortic aneurysm is a protrusion of the wall of the aorta. In severe cases hypertension can cause tearing of the artery and internal bleeding. Platelets then form clots at the site of tearing and these may break off and enter the circulation system. Aortic aneurysms are treated with a mixture of health education and health promotion aimed at reducing cardio-vascular risk factors and in serious cases surgery to repair the artery wall.

Cardiac arrhythmias

The cardiac conduction system keeps the heart beating at a steady pace. However, it is vulnerable to dysfunction, termed cardiac arrhythmia. Arrhythmias arise from irregular electrical activity which disrupts the rhythm of heart beat causing it to beat out of sequence. Cardiac arrhythmias can affect both atrial and ventricular function, causing them to work in an asymmetrical manner.

Cardiac arrhythmias can be very serious, resulting in cardiac arrest and sudden death. This occurs during fibrillation. Fibrillation is the contraction of the cardiac muscle fibres in a disorderly sequence where the chambers do not contract as a single unit which causes disruption to the pumping mechanism (Waugh and Grant 2006). However, outcomes can be non-serious where the person suffers from minor palpitations.

Causes of cardiac arrhythmias include conduction disorders (see below), lack of blood volume, for example, following a serious self-harm incident when a client may have lost blood, over active thyroid gland, adverse drug reaction and anxiety. Treatment includes anti-arrhythmia medications, fitting a pacemaker or an implantable cardioverter and defibrillator in episodes of sustained ventricular tachycardia (BHF 2005b).

Conduction disorders

Atrial fibrillation

Atrial fibrillation (AF) is an irregular heart beat that affects the atria causing the heart to pump rapidly and irregularly; approximately 46,000 new cases of AF are diagnosed in the UK every year (BHF 2007b). Table 5.2 shows the causes and symptoms of atrial fibrillation.

Treatment of atrial fibrillation

AF is usually treated by electrical cardioversion, a procedure normally done under general anaesthetic. In cardioversion a controlled electrical current is applied to the chest wall which helps to restore the heart to a normal rhythm (BHF 2007b). The current stops the heart momentarily and allows for normal cardiac conduction to be resumed. Following cardioversion

Table 5.2 Causes of and symptoms of atrial fibrillation (BHF 2007b)

Causes	Symptoms
CHD that leads to hypertension	Palpitations (an awareness of your heartbeat)
Adverse drug reaction	Feeling faint
Poor lifestyle factors	Breathlessness
Overactive thyroid gland	
Heart valve disease	
Acute lung infections such as pneumonia	
Electrolyte imbalance	

the client may need to take anti-arrhythmic drugs to keep their heart in a normal rhythm (BHF 2008a).

Clients who have had cardioversion will require close monitoring as the small shock might dislodge a clot (if one is there). To reduce the risk of secondary problems from clots, the client may be prescribed a blood thinning agent in the weeks leading up to the procedure (BHF 2008a). Close monitoring to ensure compliance is important. However, you should also educate and empower the client to adhere to treatment by explaining the significance of taking it. You should use jargon free language and encourage them to express any fears, while offering continual reassurance.

Ventricular fibrillation

Ventricular fibrillation (VF) is an extremely fast and chaotic electrical abnormality in the ventricles. It can only be diagnosed by an ECG (BHF 2005b). VF greatly impairs the heart's ability to pump blood in a coordinated way and is designated as a medical emergency (Waugh and Grant 2006). During an MI the heart is particularly vulnerable to ventricular arrhythmias which are the commonest cause of death in MI (BHF 2005b).

The only effective treatment for VF is defibrillation. Because there is no cardiac output during VF, death will result in the absence of expertly administered cardiopulmonary resuscitation (BHF 2005b).

Cardiac arrest

Cardiac arrest (CA) is defined as 'the cessation of effective pumping action of the heart, abrupt loss of consciousness, absence of pulse and breathing stops' (McFerran 2008: 77). The cardiovascular conditions outlined here will eventually lead to a CA if lifestyle behaviours are not modified or CHD is not diagnosed and treated early enough. CA may occur in mental health settings due to the following factors:

- Hypovolaemia: a decrease in blood volume in circulation, e.g. following severe cutting or frequent cutting in short periods;

Table 5.3 Causes of and symptoms of ventricular fibrillation

Causes	Symptoms
Underlying heart condition	Fainting
Genetic predisposition	Breathlessness
Brugada syndrome	Cardiac arrest

- Hypoxia: a lack of oxygen in the blood which affects the heart and other organs, e.g. following asphyxiation by hanging or during physical restraint;
- Acidosis: abnormal blood pH due to increased acidity of blood plasma, e.g. due to tricyclic antidepressant overdose, diabetic ketoacidosis, shock;
- Illicit drug use: cocaine and amphetamines are stimulants that can cause cardiac arrest.

Other coronary problems

There are a range of coronary problems but our focus here is on the most common ones. Your level of knowledge and skills will be dependent on the different types of cardiovascular problems that you encounter in practice. As you encounter more then your knowledge, skills, confidence and practice should develop.

Angina

Coronary problems may cause the heart's own blood supply to become compromised. When the heart is working with a reduced blood supply the person may experience pain or discomfort on exertion; this is called angina. Angina is an 'uncomfortable feeling or pain in the chest. It usually feels like a heaviness or tightness in the centre of the chest which may spread to the arms, neck, jaw, back or stomach' (BHF 2006: 5).

Risk factors for angina include:

- smoking
- hypertension
- high blood cholesterol level
- little physical activity
- diabetes
- being overweight or obese
- a family history

(adapted from BHF 2006)

Treatment of angina

Angina is generally treated by medication but in serious cases surgery, e.g. coronary angioplasty or a surgical bypass may be required. Drug treatment has different effects:

- Aspirin reduces the chance of blood clots developing in blood vessels that may cause angina.
- Statins help to lower cholesterol levels which can lead to atherosclerosis.
- Beta blockers reduce the heart rate by limiting the effect of adrenaline.
- Nitrates and potassium channel activators increase the blood supply to the heart.

(BHF 2006a)

Heart block

The heart's pumping mechanism is controlled by the cardiac conduction system; the AV node acting as the natural pacemaker. Heart block develops when the electrical impulses from the AV node cannot get through due to disruption. There are different degrees of heart block and treatment depends on severity.

Treatment of heart block

Heart block is usually treated by fitting a pacemaker which takes over the electrical conduction function (see BHF 2008b). Clients undergoing a pacemaker procedure will need continual support and reassurance to alleviate anxiety. Your goal is to emphasize the benefits of this treatment, give education and answer any questions in language the client understands.

Heart failure

Heart failure occurs when one of the ventricles loses its functioning. When the right ventricle fails, deoxygenated blood cannot flow to the lungs for gaseous exchange to occur. This causes congestion where there is a 'back-up' of deoxygenated blood in the circulatory system. When the left ventricle fails, oxygenated blood accumulates causing less to get pumped around the body. The danger of pooling is that blood clots can form and break off, entering the blood stream as emboli. These can cause blockage in blood vessels leading to further complications such as stroke.

Congestive cardiac failure

This occurs when there is both left and right ventricular failure with a corresponding combination of systemic and pulmonary symptoms (Webster and Thompson 2006). This is one of the most common causes of oedema where the decreased blood flow reduces the quantity of tissue fluids that can be drained away. This excess fluid then accumulates around the ankles or wrists.

Treatment of congestive cardiac failure

Depending on the severity this may entail immediate hospitalisation in a specialist coronary care unit (CCU). In this case your role will most likely be liaising with the coronary care team and observing the client to maintain their mental health status. The client will naturally be anxious as the CCU can be an anxiety provoking environment. The client will need space to ventilate their anxieties so you should be there to provide support and reassurance. Having someone familiar with them will help. You will act as a conduit between the CCU team, the client and your own team, helping to explain procedures, reasons they are needed and keeping your own team informed.

Post-operative and continuing care may also be a feature of treatment. Again you will be acting in a liaising capacity as the follow up is of a specialist nature. Your role here is to monitor physical observations and progress, including wound healing and preventing infection, if surgery has occurred. Here you may need to refresh skills of aseptic technique when changing dressings. You will also need to ensure that infection control mechanisms are in place to minimize the risk of hospital acquired infections and ensure safe disposal of clinical waste. Communicating progress with the inter-professional team will also be an important role as will supporting the client and their family/carer through the post-operative and recuperation period.

Assessing cardiovascular health in our clients

Assessing cardiovascular function is a common practice (see Chapter 3) and the most frequent ways this is done include

- pulse
- blood pressure
- blood tests
- electrocardiogram
- pulse oximetry

The key techniques that are used are

- observation
- palpation
- inspection
- pathology

Box 5.3   List some causes of chest pain.
Exercise

Observation

Assessing cardiovascular function is an important skill for practitioners given the prevalence of cardiac problems in our clients. Factors that influence assessment include the presenting problem and the approach you adopt. Therefore it is very important that you know your client, their past medical history and any significant close family history of coronary problems. From observation and a general survey we can comment on the following:

- General appearance: does the person look healthy? Do they appear overweight? Which lifestyle risk factors can you determine, e.g. smoking?
- Skin: assess colour, pallor, cyanosis, oedema, sweatiness
- Respiration: audible breathing distress, crackling, shallowness
- Mobility: uses a lot of effort, use of walking aids, requires assistance

Abnormal pulse

The most common abnormalities of pulse occur when the heart beats too fast or too slow. A pulse that is too fast, i.e. over 100 beats per minute, is referred to as tachycardia and a pulse that is too slow, i.e. under 60 beats per minute, is referred to as bradycardia (Trim 2004). See Table 5.4.

Treatment

The management and treatment of an abnormal pulse will be considered on a continuum related to the cause and the severity of the problem. This will include either/or non-invasive interventions or invasive procedures.

Tachycardia

Depending on the cause, tachycardia can be treated with lifestyle changes including those found in Table 5.5.

Table 5.4 Abnormal pulse ranges

Pulse type	Range	Characteristics	Possible cause
Tachycardia	Over 100 beats per minute	Bounding, fast, thready	History or current coronary illness, anxiety or stress, haemorrhage, side effects of medication
Normal	60–80 beats per minute	Regular and strong	
Bradycardia	Under 60 beats per minute	Weak, thready	Heart block, drug use, thyroid dysfunction, electrolyte imbalance

Table 5.5 Using lifestyle changes to treat tachycardia

Lifestyle factor	Action	Rationale
Diet	Use a balanced diet – reduce fat and salt intake and increase fruit and fibre	A diet high in fat and salt contributes to the development of CHD; reducing intake of these will help lower blood lipid levels
Substance Use	Stop smoking, or at least restrict tobacco use Reduce alcohol use	Smoking is a factor in development of atherosclerosis and respiratory disorders Alcohol use is a factor in CHD
Activity	Increase physical activity	Helps to reduce obesity through controlled weight loss, increases cardiovascular functioning and can also improve self-esteem

In cases where clinical interventions are required, tachycardia can be treated with anti-arrhythmic and antihypertensive medications. These medications will help lower blood pressure by aiding vasodilation and reducing sodium retention. In severe cases cardioversion may be required.

Bradycardia

When the heart beats slowly blood flow decreases. Blood may pool in the heart and a clot may form which can lead to an embolism. This increases the risk of pulmonary embolism, stroke or blockage of smaller blood vessels in the extremities, e.g. the legs, leading to ulcers. Depending on cause and severity, bradycardia can be treated by giving anti-coagulation drugs to prevent clotting or treating any underlying electrolyte imbalance or thyroid problem. In some cases a pacemaker may be needed to help the heart beat regularly.

Garden (2005) outlines the significance of the pulse measurement in a specific mental health context (see Table 5.6). You should use the table to contextualize the importance of pulse measurement in any of your clients who might come under the 'potential association' column.

Hypertension

Hypertension is a persistently high blood pressure (BP) and is a common problem. It is diagnosed when the average of three different BP readings, taken at rest, on three different days over a period of time, e.g. 2 or 3 weeks, are compared. To confirm the diagnosis an ECG will be required. If BP is only slightly elevated, repeated measurements should be obtained over several months, because there is often a regression to normal levels (European Society of Hypertension 2003). Further diagnostic tests may be required, e.g. cholesterol levels, blood glucose levels and urinalysis to determine if there is blood or protein in the urine which may be indicative of kidney damage due to hypertension (BF 2005: 12).

In over 9 out of every 10 people there is no definite cause of high blood pressure (BHF 2005a: 10). However, in our client group we know that lifestyle factors and adverse drug reactions can contribute to it. When assessing blood pressure it is useful to have a recommended guideline that can increase the evidence base of clinical practice. Table 5.7 would be a welcome addition to clinical decision-making processes.

Other factors in cardiovascular assessment

Taking physical observations is a direct way of estimating cardiovascular function. However, there are other ways in which we can perceive problems. A general survey may indicate the presence of risk factors that can contribute to development of CHD. Therefore, if a client does

Table 5.6 Significance of pulse in mental health

Sign	Potential association
Tachycardia	Infection, autonomic arousal/stress, neuroleptic malignant syndrome
Bradycardia	Clozapine therapy, hypothyroidism, tricyclic antidepressants
Atrial fibrillation	Hyperthyroidism, vascular dementia
Arrhythmias	Tricyclic antidepressants, antipsychotics, lithium

Source: Garden 2005 reproduced with permission from the Royal College of Psychiatrists

Table 5.7 British Hypertension Society classifications of blood pressure levels

Category	Systolic blood pressure (mmHg)	Diastolic blood pressure (mmHg)
Optimal blood pressure	≥ 120	≥ 80
Normal blood pressure	≥ 130	≥ 85
High-normal blood pressure	130–139	85–89
Grade 1 hypertension (mild)	140–159	90–99
Grade 2 hypertension (moderate)	160–179	100–109
Grade 3 hypertension (severe)	≥ 180	≥ 110
Isolated systolic hypertension (Grade 1)	140–159	≥ 90
Isolated systolic hypertension (Grade 2)	≥ 160	≥ 90

Source: Williams *et al.* 2004: 142, reproduced with the permission from the British Hypertension Society

not currently have it (represented by a stable pulse and blood pressure) failure to modify the risk factors will inevitably lead to the risk of developing CHD.

Other physiological signs

- Skin colour: flushed and red indicating vasodilation or cyanosed and blue indicating lack of blood supply. Cyanosis will render the extremities cold to touch which you might notice when taking the pulse.
- Temperature: increased temperature will increase blood pressure and indicate signs of infection. Temperature recording usually accompanies blood pressure, pulse and respiration as part of the 'baseline obs'.
- Respiration: laboured or distressed breathing may also indicate a cardiovascular problem. In emergency situations this will be extremely noticeable and you will have to act quickly to prevent deterioration.
- Oedema: this is excess fluid retained by the body and may be present in the wrists or ankles. A quick inspection and palpation (pressing the raised area) will indicate the extent of fluid retention. Oedema requires further investigation as it indicates a cardiovascular or renal problem, especially in clients taking lithium. A diuretic may be prescribed to alleviate fluid retention.
- Dizziness: clients reporting episodes of dizziness or light-headedness when rising may be experiencing orthostatic hypotension. You should ask by way of a general question if they have experienced such symptoms.
- Waist size: a useful risk indicator for CHD. A waist size over 35 inches in women and 40 inches in men is associated with increased risk of high blood pressure, type 2 diabetes, dyslipidaemia and metabolic syndrome (Janssen *et al.* 2002).
- BMI: an important indicator as BP rises with rising BMI (Wild and Byrne 2006) who go on to

report that a US study showed high blood pressure was the most common condition related to overweight and obesity.

Box 5.4   How can we reduce the risks of cardiovascular illness in our client group?
Exercise

Using health promotion with clients with CHD

In terms of health promotion there are three ways in which we can tackle the problem of cardiovascular illness. By far the best way of managing it is by preventing it. Here your role will be primary prevention – preventing the development of cardiovascular illness by screening for signs and symptoms of heart problems or other conditions such as obesity and diabetes.

In a position statement 'Lifestyle changes in managing hypertension' (European Society of Hypertension 2003) a consensus in lifestyle factors that can serve in primary prevention include:

- smoking cessation
- weight reduction
- reduction of excessive alcohol intake
- physical exercise
- reduction of salt intake
- increase in fruit and vegetable intake, and
- decrease in saturated and total fat intake.

Secondary prevention concerns the management of the early stages of conditions, reducing their impact on the client's health and well-being. For cardiovascular illness, medications such as statins are prescribed to lower cholesterol in conjunction with primary prevention measures outlined above. Your role will be preventing further deterioration in physical health by

- encouraging compliance with medications and dietary regimes;
- supporting clients in changing behaviours, e.g. beginning to exercise;
- if trained – providing smoking cessation interventions or referral to smoking cessation services.

Tertiary prevention is designed to increase the quality of life of people with long term conditions that require active treatment. This stage is more advanced than primary or secondary prevention and may consist of invasive interventions such as cardiac surgery which will require intensive aftercare.

Care planning

The nursing process remains the main care planning framework. Roper, Logan and Tierney's (1996) Activities of Daily Living is a familiar model which can structure our care plans. Our role in care planning will depend on the severity of the problem. However, we need to practise safely and within our competence. Complex conditions will require us to liaise between teams and adopt a monitoring, evaluating and reporting role. We may take on a shared care coordinator role for less complex problems where we plan and provide care in a multi-professional team. Whatever our role, care planning activity will need to be safe, competent and evidence based.

Treating and managing CHD

Daniels (2002) lists the clinical priorities for managing CHD as

- Normalizing blood pressure
- Correcting hyperlipidaemia
- Controlling diabetes
- Controlling clotting disorders if present
- Reducing weight if overweight/obese
- Lifestyle modification priorities involve smoking cessation, regular physical activity and the consumption of a healthy diet.

Table 5.8 provides an illustration of factors that you might consider when care planning for someone with a coronary problem using Roper, Logan and Tierney's Model (1996). This is a

Table 5.8 Factors to consider when care planning for someone with a coronary problem

Activity of daily living	Example of care planning activity
1 Maintaining a safe environment	This might relate to homeostasis of the internal body environment. We can achieve this through • monitoring baseline observations • monitoring physical interventions such as medications • evaluating the effectiveness of treatment • re-visiting care plan if condition deteriorates Physical environment is also important as limiting physical exertion when moving around is necessary. Adapting the home environment to minimize levels of exertion and promote independence and mobility, e.g. installation of stair lift, adapting showers, toilet seats and installing hand rails.
2 Breathing	Monitoring respirations is a core observation as breathlessness is a clinical feature of coronary problems. Breathlessness can be anxiety provoking due to the associated discomfort and its role as a reinforcing agent of illness. Respirations should also be monitored during sleep. Observations and interventions include • respiration rate • pulse oximetry • oxygen therapy • posture when sitting or lying • collecting sputum samples for pathology and assessing any cough
3 Communicating	Care planning and treatment for cardiovascular conditions can be very complex. Any instructions or explanations should be • jargon free • easy to understand • the subject of regular feedback to ensure comprehension, and clarification that things have been understood You should also give reassurance to alleviate anxiety. Encourage clients to ventilate feelings and develop psychological coping strategies, or acceptance of the condition. This will decrease anxiety as they find they can still have a social life as long as they are not over exerting the heart.
4 Mobilizing	While encouraging fitness is important this should not be too strenuous. Set small and safe targets, e.g. • involving physiotherapy to develop an exercise plan • walking short distances gradually increasing this

Table 5.8 continued

	• considering relaxation therapy to help the resting process and cope with stress
	• encouraging the client to rise slowly to prevent dizziness and light headedness
	• encouraging rest also

(Also refer to maintaining a safe environment above.)

5 Eating and drinking	Diet may need to change. If it does not problems may deteriorate. A dietician can advise on nutrition.

• reduce calorie intake in obese clients
• encourage fruit and fibre
• introduce a low salt diet
• reduce salt intake, e.g. encourage no salt at the table but small quantities when cooking, consider low salt alternatives
• reduce/abstain from alcohol intake
• reduce caffeine intake

Occupational therapy can help develop cooking skills.

6 Eliminating	• record fluid balance if required
	• encourage adequate hydration
	• monitor blood electrolyte levels
	• prevent constipation to reduce risk of straining on elimination

7 Personal cleansing and dressing	Promote independence here to illustrate that the client can still function.

• ensure safety when bathing/showering as this can be tiring
• use shower seat aids to minimize exertion
• observe skin integrity – reduced blow flow and oedema may compromise skin so avoid rough towelling/drying following bathing
• use a moisturiser on dry, flaky skin to help recovery

8 Maintaining body temperature	• monitor body temperature to observe for any infection
	• encourage appropriate attire

9 Working and playing	• as for mobilizing above
	• time off work may be required for those who are employed
	• recreational activities may have to be less strenuous initially
	• explore local self-help or support groups that might have social activities

10 Sleeping	• observe for sleep difficulties relating to respiration
	• use of extra pillows to assist breathing
	• discourage sleeping during the day
	• consider medication if required

11 Expressing sexuality	• depending on the severity of the problem sexual activity may decrease initially
	• explain this to the client as for working and playing above
	• reassure that usual sexual activity will return

12 Dying	Clients may be preoccupied with death or dying

• allow clients to express fears
• reassure that with treatment and lifestyle changes life can still be enjoyed
• discuss fears of the future openly and discourage catastrophic thinking
• encourage joining a support group to get peer support

general outline as there are just too many individual factors to cover in a case story. Our aim is to restore normal constant heart function or as close as can be, given cardiac muscle damage.

Medications used to treat coronary heart problems

There are many types of medications that can be prescribed in the treatment and management of heart problems. It is important that you are familiar with those prescribed to your client group and both their desired and undesired effects. These medications can be taken in various forms and you should be aware of this in order to prevent maladministration. This is also an important factor for client education – that they are aware of the route of administration when they are self-medicating. This part of the chapter will give a quick guide to common medications. However, you will need to do some extra reading in this area yourself.

Drug treatment has different effects:

- Agents 'thin' the blood reducing its viscosity, decreasing risk of blood clots.
- Agents reduce the heart rate to lower blood pressure.
- Agents cause vasodilation which increases blood supply to the heart.
- Agents reduce the risk of coronary problems by lowering cholesterol.

There are seven possible routes of administration for coronary medications:

- orally: swallowed via mouth
- sublingually: medication is dissolved under the tongue
- spray: the medication is sprayed under the tongue
- patch: a patch is placed on the arm and medication slowly released (similar principle to nicotine patches)
- subcutaneously: injection under the skin (dermis and epidermis)
- intramuscularly: injection into a muscle
- intravenously: directly into a vein

Alpha blockers

Alpha blockers are vasodilators which reduce vasoconstriction. Vasodilation helps to increase blood flow to the heart.

Beta blockers

Beta blockers are drugs that block the actions of the sympathetic nervous system by reducing the levels of the hormone adrenaline, which increases heart rate. They are used to help prevent attacks of angina, to lower blood pressure, to help control abnormal heart rhythms, and to reduce the risk of a further heart attack in people who have already had one. They are sometimes also used in heart failure (BHF 2007c).

ACE inhibitors

ACE inhibitors are used to treat hypertension by lowering BP. They have a vasodilator action and also reduce sodium retention. The most significant side effect is a persistent, dry, irritating cough (BHF 2007c). Kidney function should also be monitored as these drugs can affect the renal system, especially in clients taking lithium.

Calcium channel blockers

Calcium causes the cells of the heart to contract or the blood vessels to narrow. This restricts blood flow and oxygen levels. Calcium channel blockers reduce calcium so that the heart and blood vessels can dilate. This causes diastole, the 'resting phase' of the heart's pumping cycle, to last longer (BHF 2007c). This reduces blood pressure by reducing heart rate which will help clients with angina.

Diuretics

These help with the treatment of oedema by reducing sodium levels and increasing fluid loss.

Loop diuretics

This type of diuretic prevents re-absorption of fluids in the kidney, specifically the loop of Henle.

Statins

High cholesterol levels are a risk factor for atherosclerosis. Statins work in two ways: they reduce the amount of cholesterol produced by the liver and they stimulate the removal of low density lipoproteins (LDL) from circulation back to the liver (Evered 2007). LDL is termed 'bad' cholesterol as it sticks to the artery wall leading to atheroma.

Blood thinning agents

Drugs such as warfarin, heparin and aspirin help reduce the risk of blood clots forming.

Box 5.5 Exercise	List the medications for cardiovascular illness currently taken by your clients.

Orthostatic hypotension

Orthostatic hypotension (OH), also known as postural hypotension, is a sudden drop in blood pressure (25mmHg systolic or 10mmHg diastolic) when the client moves from a horizontal to a vertical position (Smith *et al.* 2008). It is a common condition in individuals with cardiac problems and is an adverse drug reaction in some psychotropics. This is a key rationale for having skills in assessing and monitoring cardiovascular health. Lying and standing blood pressure is recommended in patients who are older, have diabetes or symptoms suggestive of postural hypotension (British Hypotension Society 2006).

Mathias and Kimber (1999) give a comprehensive overview of causes of postural hypotension and particular factors that we should note include

- Low blood volume
- Myocarditis
- Drug/alcohol use
- Anorexia nervosa
- Diabetes insipidus and mellitus
- Chronic renal failure
- Autonomic failure in Parkinson's disease

Other factors that relate to our clients include adverse drug reactions following treatment with antipsychotics, tricyclic antidepressants or benzodiazepines, and bulimia where there is excessive vomiting.

Symptoms of orthostatic hypotension

Symptoms of OH include

- dizziness or being 'light-headed'
- feeling faint
- weakness in the legs

When someone gets up too quickly they may feel dizzy, nauseous or faint and may even lose consciousness. Loss of consciousness presents other potential risks such as head injury. Clients who take medication that risks OH should have regular blood pressure and pulse recorded. They should also be asked specific questions relating to symptoms of OH as they may put symptoms down to natural causes such as the ageing process. A client group more vulnerable to OH are clients in care of older people services, as the natural ageing process can contribute to it. They should be monitored regularly.

Treatment of OH

Mathias and Kimber (1999) suggest that treatment can be divided into three categories which can be a useful guide for interventions when care planning:

- Things to be avoided, e.g. sudden head-up postural change (especially on waking), high environmental temperature (including hot baths), large meals (especially with refined carbohydrate).
- Things to be introduced, e.g. small, frequent meals, judicious exercise (including swimming).
- Things to be considered, e.g. elastic stockings, pharmacological measures such as erythropoietin.

Care planning for OH

The treatment of OH will depend on the severity and a care plan will be required. As OH is not an uncommon adverse drug reaction we should be able to write a competent and safe care plan. The uncertainty surrounding staff skills and responsibilities for physical care may mean that care plans such as this may be best drawn up in an inter-professional context utilizing the expertise of doctors and a specialist cardiac nurse practitioner.

Box 5.6 Case example

John has developed OH as a result of his antipsychotic medications. He complains of feeling dizzy at times. He asks his primary nurse for some advice. Ruben sits with John and together they develop a care plan (see Table 5.9).

Table 5.9 Ruben and John's care plan

Activity of daily living	Example of care planning activity
1 Maintaining a safe environment	The internal body environment will be monitored through • baseline observations – Ruben explains that blood pressure has to be monitored both lying and standing to assess extent of change • monitoring physical interventions such as medications • evaluating the effectiveness of treatment • revisiting care plan if condition deteriorates Physical environment will be modified to assist with rising and standing, e.g. high backed chairs, toilet handles
2 Breathing	Breathing should also be monitored: • respiration rate • posture when sitting or lying • stop smoking – refer to smoking cessation specialist and use nicotine replacement aids
3 Communicating	Care planning and treatment for OH should be explained in a way John can understand in particular when he needs to follow instructions: • jargon free • seek regular feedback to ensure comprehension and • clarification that things have been understood Psychological – Ruben should reassure John as to his physical well-being. He gives John appropriate explanations of what has been happening and reassures him that it can be effectively managed.
4 Mobilizing	Ruben should ensure John's safety by • encouraging John to rise slowly to prevent dizziness and light headedness • on rising he suggests John pauses momentarily to further prevent dizziness • for safety Ruben suggests John uses various aids when mobilizing (Also refer to maintaining a safe environment above.)
5 Eating and drinking	Diet may need to change. If it does not problems may deteriorate. • monitor salt intake (salt intake in line with recommended levels – 6mg per day, DH 2006) • reduce/abstain from alcohol intake • caffeine intake may need to be reduced • refrain from eating large meals Occupational therapy can help with cooking skills.
6 Eliminating	• record fluid balance with an input output chart • encourage adequate hydration • take bloods to monitor electrolytes • prevent constipation by encouraging adequate hydration and fibre intake to reduce risk of straining on elimination
7 Personal cleansing and dressing	• promote independence in this domain to illustrate to John that he can still complete activities • ensure safety when bathing, suggest a shower rather than a bath from where he has to stand up • use a shower seat to minimize exertion • encourage not to stand for long periods, e.g. when shaving John should sit down

(Continued Overleaf)

Table 5.9 Continued

Activity of daily living	Example of care planning activity
8 Maintaining body temperature	• Excessive heat may lead to OH
9 Working and playing	• As for mobilizing above • Explore local self-help or support groups that might have social activities
10 Sleeping	• Use of extra pillows to assist in better posture • Ensure safety when rising from bed

Summary of key points

Cardiac problems will affect three key areas:

- the pumping mechanism: atrial and ventricle weakness, heart valve weakness;
- the cardiac conduction system: cardiac arrhythmias, fibrillation;
- the vascular network: total or partial blood vessel blockage, thrombosis.

The prevalence of cardiovascular problems is not well understood in our clients. However, we know that our clients face the same risk factors (apart from psychotropic medication) for coronary problems as the general population but are more likely to die from them.

It is important that practitioners have an understanding of the cardiovascular system so that they can recognize signs and symptoms of illness and respond effectively. Practitioners must also recognize the value of liaising with the inter-professional team and specialist nurses for help and support and should suggest that their managers support them in this.

Finally, practitioners should be aware of safety issues in planning care for people with coronary problems. This will include their knowledge of the desired and undesired effects of medications – those for treating the mental health problem and those for treating the coronary problem.

Quick quiz

1 Define tachycardia.
2 Define bradycardia.
3 What are the stages of the cardiac cycle?
4 Define the terms 'systolic' and 'diastolic'.
5 Describe blood flow through the heart.

Assessing respiratory health in mental health

By the end of this chapter you will have:

- Outlined the structure and function of the respiratory system
- Defined key terms in respiration
- Explored respiratory conditions prevalent in our clients
- Explored the impact of smoking on respiratory health
- Explored the difference between routine and emergency respiratory assessment
- Examined treatment and management of respiratory conditions
- Examined aspects of care planning and management of breathlessness

Box 6.1
Exercise
List the factors that affect respiratory function.

Introduction

Q: Do your client's cough?
A: (Laugh) yes, they cough all the time.
Q: Why do they cough?
A: Because they smoke.

This is a regular exchange I have when teaching physical health issues. While it appears logical that clients cough because they smoke, this rationale may undervalue the cough as a clinical symptom due to its perceived 'usualness'. Practitioners may see smoking as a personal characteristic of the client rather than a risk factor for respiratory disorders. This may reduce the inclination to offer smoking cessation or health promotion because smoking is part of the person's life.

Research has established some very important statistics concerning smoking in our client group. Our clients have higher death rates from respiratory disorders with a SMR 250 (Harris and Barraclough 1998) and a greater smoking prevalence: Brown *et al.* (1999) found between 62 and 81 per cent of people with SMI smoke tobacco compared with 25 per cent of the general population. The prevalence of smoking among the UK adult population was 22 per cent in 2006 (Goddard 2006) but studies show rates as high as 80 per cent among people with schizophrenia (McNeill 2001), and more than half (52 per cent) of schizophrenic smokers living in institutions wanted to give up smoking (McNeill 2001). The prevalence of respiratory conditions remains largely unknown in our client population. In a US study, Himelhoch *et al.* (2004) surveyed a random sample of 200 clients to estimate the prevalence of COPD. They found the following in relation to smoking and respiratory illness in their client sample:

- Smoking prevalence: 60.5 per cent (22 per cent nationally)
- COPD prevalence: 22.6 per cent (5 per cent in the general population)
- Chronic bronchitis: 19.6 per cent
- Emphysema: 7.5 per cent
- Asthma: 18.5 per cent
- Asthma and COPD: 33.3 per cent

Risk factors affecting respiratory function

Risk factors for respiratory disorders can be categorized as

- demographic factors – social class, occupational factors;
- lifestyle factors – smoking, illicit drug use, alcohol abuse;
- psychological factors – anxiety disorders, panic attacks;
- physiological factors – genetic disorders, allergies, neck or chest trauma, diagnosed respiratory disorders;
- medications – some antipsychotics may cause cough and nasal congestion.

Reasons for respiratory disorders in people with mental illness

Smoking is the main factor for the high prevalence of respiratory problems. It is the most significant public health concern in mental health as it causes and contributes to high mortality and morbidity. We need to have competent skills in assessing respiratory health, identifying respiratory illnesses and care planning for respiratory care. Liaison with primary care services will be a key role for community practitioners.

Harris and Barraclough (1998) also note higher mortality rates for infectious diseases in our clients. Adverse drug reactions can lead to a decrease in white blood cells which may compromise the immune system, leaving clients more vulnerable to opportunistic chest infections (see Chapter 8). Clients on these medications should be offered appropriate immunizations as a high risk group.

Anatomy and physiology of the respiratory system

The respiratory system has two distinct tracts, which is helpful when considering which part is affected during a respiratory assessment (see Figure 6.1). The upper respiratory tract consists of the mouth, nose, pharynx and larynx while the lower respiratory tract contains the trachea, lungs, bronchi, bronchioles, alveoli, pulmonary capillary network and pleural membranes (Kozier *et al.* 2008a). As with the heart, the lungs have pleural membranes which keep them in place and this contains a lubricant which allows for painless breathing.

The respiratory system is responsible for

- warming and filtering inhaled air for foreign particles;
- control of breathing;
- enabling ventilation;

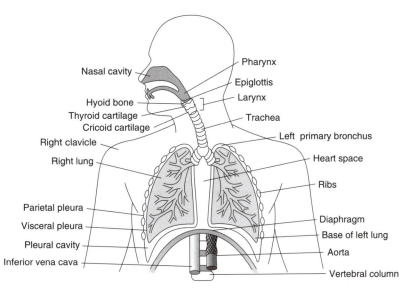

Figure 6.1 The respiratory system

- expelling carbon dioxide;
- maintaining blood gas homeostasis.

In homeostasis there is a balance between oxygen and carbon dioxide levels in the blood. However, if an imbalance occurs, for example, too much carbon dioxide, then chemoreceptors located in the aorta and carotid arteries detect this. They send a message to the medulla oblongata (control centre) which instructs the lungs to increase respiration to increase oxygen intake. The respiratory system increases respiration rate until homeostasis is restored. The feedback loop then completes the cycle and breathing returns to normal.

How the lungs work

Respiration is an involuntary reflex involving ventilation. Ventilation involves inspiration – air flow into the lungs – and expiration – air flow out of the lungs (Kozier 2008). This is what we measure in baseline respirations. When air enters the mouth and nose it is warmed and filtered by tiny hairs, cilia, which remove any foreign particles.

When we inspire our lungs inflate. The diaphragm flattens and the inter-costal muscles allow our rib cage to expand and fill with oxygen. When we expire our lungs deflate and we expel carbon dioxide. Diffusion is a process that governs respiration. Here particles from an area of high concentration move to an area of low concentration. In respiration oxygen diffuses into the blood stream and carbon dioxide diffuses out (see Figure 6.2).

Box 6.2 **Exercise**	How does smoking affect the respiratory system?

There are two types of respiration. External respiration is the diffusion of oxygen and carbon dioxide between the alveoli and the blood in the lungs. Internal respiration occurs at a cellular

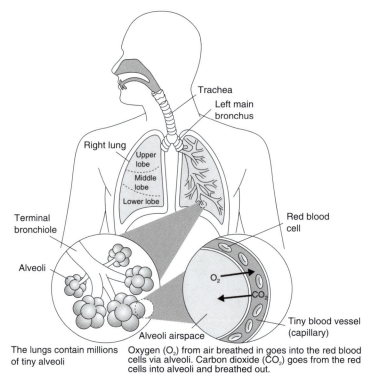

Figure 6.2 Alveoli and the process of gaseous exchange

level with diffusion of oxygen and carbon dioxide between the blood and cells. The alveoli contain white blood cells (alveolar macrophages) which keep them free from bacteria. These will attack and destroy foreign bodies which evade the cilia and enter the lungs. However, smoking inhibits the actions of the cilia and alveolar macrophages, reducing their effectiveness, which is a reason why smokers are vulnerable to frequent chest infections.

Key terms in respiration

The significance of respiration for mental health practitioners

Our clients smoke significantly more than the general population and are likely to die earlier from respiratory disorders. Knowledge of respiratory function is important in identifying respiratory problems accurately, so that appropriate treatment can be given. Practitioners working with socially excluded groups, for example, homeless people, who face significant challenges around communicable diseases such as TB, which will be explored further in this chapter.

With many countries now adopting no smoking policies in public places, there is a significant challenge for practitioners to meet this public health agenda. Clients are also being challenged to change their smoking habits. Practitioners should enable clients to stop smoking by engaging and supporting them in smoking cessation and nicotine replacement therapy.

Table 6.1 Key terms in respiration adapted from Jevon and Ewens (2001)

Characteristic	Presentation	Possible cause
Dyspnoea	Shortness of breath	Asthma, COPD
Tachypnoea	Increased respiratory rate	Anxiety, post-exercise
Bradypnoea	Abnormally slow respiratory rate	Hypothermia
Orthopnoea	Breathlessness when lying flat	CHD, COPD
Cheyne-Stokes	Alternating periods of apnoea and hyperpnoea	Observed in people at end stage of life
Kussmal breathing	Also referred to as 'air hunger', characterized by deep, rapid, gasping/gulping respirations	Metabolic acidosis, renal failure, hypovolaemia
Hyperventilation	Rapid ventilation presenting as extreme breathlessness	Anxiety disorders
Haemoptysis	Expectoration of blood from the respiratory tract	Chest trauma, tumour, exposure to occupational hazard, e.g. asbestos
Hypoxia	Decrease in oxygen supply to the tissues and cells	Hypovolaemia, asphyxiation

Smoking

Smoking is a lifestyle factor and the second major cause of death in the world (around 5 million yearly; WHO 2008d). In the European Union, tobacco is the single largest cause of avoidable death accounting for over a million deaths (European Commission 2002) while in the UK, 106,000 people die from smoking-related disease every year (Chief Medical Officer 2004)

Table 6.2 illustrates the public health concern regarding smoking in respect to the general population and more specifically, mental health.

Effects of smoking on the body

Smoking related disorders include cancers of the lung, mouth and oesophagus. Smoking is a prime cause of COPD and it increases the risk of atherosclerosis which leads to cardiovascular conditions such as CHD and stroke.

Cigarettes contain nicotine and Cancer Research UK (Nov 2006) reports the following:

- Nicotine is a stimulant that increases heart rate.
- Nicotine is addictive and causes withdrawal symptoms such as cravings, irritability, anxiety, difficulty concentrating, restlessness and disturbed sleep.
- Cigarette smoke contains at least 69 cancer-causing chemicals as well as other poisons like hydrogen cyanide and carbon monoxide.

Why is smoking more prevalent in mental health care?

From a social perspective, smoking is more prevalent in lower socio-economic groups, where our clients usually come from. Between 1991 and 1993, among men aged 20 to 64 in professional work, 17 in every 100,000 died of lung cancer, compared with 82 per 100,000 in unskilled manual work (DH 1998).

From a biological perspective an addiction model explains smoking behaviour. Nicotine is addictive, so when nicotine levels fall below a certain level in the blood smokers experience

Table 6.2 Comparison of general population and mental health service users smoking rates

Country	Prevalence of smoking in the general population % (WHO 2004b)	Prevalence of smoking in clients
USA	23.6	52% out-patients, 88% schizophrenia, 70% mania (Hughes et al. 1986)
UK	26.5	80% schizophrenia (McNeill 2001)
Australia	19.5	39% of people with a mental illness, 90% schizophrenia (Access Economics 2007)

unpleasant withdrawal symptoms which are relieved by smoking. This develops into a cycle of smoking to relieve withdrawal symptoms.

Clients may use smoking as a coping mechanism for stress and anxiety. However, this self-medication hypothesis has not been proven. People may feel that smoking relieves their stress or anxiety but this might be conflated with the addiction model. The symptoms of nicotine withdrawal cause anxiety and stress so smoking relieves withdrawal, hence it relieves anxiety and stress.

Self-medication may be considered in relation to schizophrenia. Levin and Rezvani (2000) found evidence that nicotine has an effect in both reversing the adverse effects of antipsychotic drugs and the cognitive impairment of schizophrenia itself. Furthermore, Patkar et al. (2002) found a link between nicotine dependence and negative symptoms in people with schizophrenia. This study also showed that duration of illness and alcohol use also predicted smoking.

The reality for many clients is less scientifically glamorous with boredom at institutional life reported as a key factor in smoking (McNeil 2004). Smoking is often seen as a 'way of life' for clients, a way to socialize or pass time by. In a survey of patients in a UK medium secure unit 84 per cent reported that they smoked (Micklejohn 2003).

I believe it is the culture of acceptance of smoking in mental health rather than a culture of smoking that is the simplest answer. Smoking is an activity that is highly tolerated by practitioners. Indeed Gubbay's 1992 research showed that mental health nurses have a higher prevalence of smoking than other nurses. We may even use smoking as a means of calming clients or socializing with them. Trying to introduce change can be met with intolerance and fatalist attitudes, e.g. 'you can't teach an old dog new tricks'. Indeed cigarettes are often used in ad hoc token economy systems in psychiatric units (Nash 2008).

Smoking and psychotropic medications

Nicotine stimulates the release of dopamine (Mental Health Foundation 2007). An increase in dopamine is a biological theory of psychosis. Smoking can increase the rate at which psychotropic medication is metabolized in the body. This means that drugs pass through the body quicker. Therefore higher doses of medications may be required for heavy smokers.

Desai et al. (2001) found that smoking is associated with increased clearance of benzodiazepines such as lorazepam and diazepam and antipsychotics such as haloperidol and olanzapine. Furthermore they state that plasma concentrations of chlorpromazine and clozapine are reduced by cigarette smoking. Dratcu et al. (2007) suggest that smoking and excessive caffeine use is associated with poor therapeutic responses to clozapine and should be considered in pharmacological management. There have been reports that clozapine can reduce smoking (Combs and Advokat 2000). The mechanism for this is unclear. It may be a genuine psychopharmacological action of reducing craving, or clozapine may stabilize mental state so that health promotion advice can be acted upon.

It is also important to consider the effect that smoking cessation may have on adverse drug reactions. If smokers require higher doses of medication, if they stop smoking they may suffer from adverse effects. Subsequently, as clients abstain from smoking, treatment regimes may require altering. Therefore taking a smoking history is important for both respiratory assessment and informing prescribing practices.

Smoking and illicit substances

For some clients smoking might involve illicit substances. In anecdotal accounts colleagues working in substance misuse report clients using bronchodilators prior to smoking heroin as this increases the 'hit', or clients smoking benzodiazepine 'splifs'. Respiratory complications due to substance use and smoking are illustrated in Table 6.3.

Box 6.3
Exercise   List the barriers to and opportunities for your clients stopping smoking.

Disorders of the respiratory system

Disorders of the respiratory system stem primarily from inflammation and infection. Smoking is a significant contributor to both of these, causing upper and lower respiratory tract damage and reducing the body's defences. Respiratory problems can be divided into two broad types:

* Restrictive problems occur when an individual cannot inhale a normal amount of air, e.g. due to a trauma or infection.
* Obstructive problems occur when something obstructs the flow of air into or out of the lungs, e.g. asthma, COPD, tumour.

Table 6.3 Effects of smoking illicit substances

Substance	Potential effect
Cannabis	Similar symptoms to COPD
Cocaine	Snorting leads to ulceration of nasal mucosa Necrosis and infection of nasal tissue Acute and chronic sinusitis
Crack cocaine	Smoking crack leads to acute lung injury, e.g. asthma of varying degrees Barotrauma – where drug sharing under air pressure causes rupture of the connective tissue or pleura, pulmonary oedema, alveolar haemorrhage, non-specific pneumonitis, inflammation of the bronchioles and surrounding tissues, haemoptysis, thermal injury to the lungs (due to heat of substance)
Heroin	Similar effects to inhaling cocaine vapour Acts as a respiratory depressant which can be fatal
Solvents	Hypoxia with airway obstruction Central respiratory depression Respiratory failure

Source: Adapted from Rayner and Prigmore (2008)

Lung cancer

More than 34,000 people die from lung cancer in the UK each year (Cancer UK 2008). However, the reality is that many more are suffering from debilitating smoking related disorders. Smoking is a significant cause of lung cancer. The risk of developing lung cancer is affected by level of consumption and duration of smoking (Doll *et al.* 2005), which places our clients in a high risk group.

There are two types of lung cancer:

- Small cell carcinomas account for approximately 20–25 per cent of all lung cancers (Le Pechoux *et al.* 2004).
- Non small cell lung cancer accounts for approximately 80 per cent of all lung cancers (National Institute for Health Research 2007).

Diagnosing lung cancer

The signs and symptoms of lung cancer are very similar to those of other respiratory disorders making it difficult to diagnose. Therefore by the time diagnosis is confirmed the cancer may have metastasized (spread to other sites). If this occurs the outcomes for the client are significantly worse. Diagnostic procedures for lung cancer include

- Chest x-ray
- Bronchoscopy
- Computed tomography (CT scan)
- Positron emission tomography (PET scan)

(Hunt 2008)

However, the National Collaborating Centre for Acute Care (2005) recommend urgent referral for a chest X-ray when a patient presents with haemoptysis, or any of the following unexplained or persistent (that is, lasting more than 3 weeks) symptoms or signs:

- Cough
- Chest/shoulder pain
- Dyspnoea
- Weight loss
- Chest signs
- Hoarseness
- Finger clubbing
- Features suggestive of metastasis from a lung cancer (for example in brain, bone, liver or skin)
- Cervical/supraclavicular lymphadenopathy

Our role in the diagnostic process is a screening one. As nurses spend more time with clients we should be observing changes to respiratory function. When we notice something peculiar we should assess, document and report it. If it comes to nothing, fine: it is still good practice. However, if it is something, prompt intervention can be the difference in client outcome.

Treatment

The treatment of lung cancer will depend on the specific type and the severity. Radiotherapy and chemotherapy are the main treatment methods. However, invasive surgery to remove a lung, or part of, may also be considered. Your role in this treatment will be supportive. You will act as liaison between the specialist practitioners and the mental health team. You will monitor the client's health and response to treatment through baseline observations and will also liaise with the cancer specialist nurse in respect to specific aspects of care, for example, the management of nausea following treatment.

A cancer diagnosis can be a devastating life event. Psychological support and education for both client and family will be important considerations. You will monitor mental state especially for signs of depression and hopelessness while co-monitoring the physical condition with the cancer specialist nurse. In the event that palliative care is required you will reassure the client and their family that physical suffering will be minimized through a client centred pain relief management plan. You would also arrange for spiritual support as per the client's wishes.

Chronic obstructive pulmonary disease

Chronic obstructive pulmonary disease (COPD) is a condition characterized by airflow obstruction that is usually progressive, not fully reversible and does not change markedly over several months (NICE 2004). COPD is the internationally recognized term for chronic bronchitis, emphysema, chronic obstructive airways disease, chronic airflow limitation, chronic obstructive lung disease and chronic airflow obstruction (Booker 2005). It is estimated that nearly 900,000 people in the UK have COPD but half as many again are thought to be living with it undiagnosed (NCCCC 2004). The UK Department of Health (2006a) estimates mortality from COPD at 30,000 deaths annually.

Pathophysiology of COPD

Airway obstruction is caused by excess mucous build up, inflammation, irritation or infection. This causes the airways to narrow restricting airflow. COPD is a progressive disorder where there is a loss of alveolar function. As function deteriorates there is only partial diffusion, so not all air is expelled from the lungs. This creates dead space where reduced gaseous exchange occurs. Dead space decreases lung capacity leaving less space for oxygen to occupy on respiration. This results in hypoxia which leads to tissue death.

Diagnosing COPD

There is no single diagnostic test for COPD. Diagnosis depends on clinical judgement based on a combination of history, physical examination and confirmation of the presence of airflow obstruction using spirometry (NICE 2004). However, a diagnosis of COPD should be considered in patients over the age of 35 who have a risk factor (generally smoking) and who present with one or more of the symptoms shown in Table 6.4.

Spirometry is used to test lung function and diagnose conditions such as COPD. Like PEFR (see

Table 6.4 Diagnosing COPD

Primary factors	Other factors
Chronic cough	Effort intolerance
Exertional breathlessness	Waking at night
Regular sputum production	Ankle swelling
Frequent winter 'bronchitis'	Fatigue
Wheeze	Occupational hazards
Weight loss	Chest pain
	Haemoptysis

Source: NICE (2004)

Chapter 3, pp. 104–6), spirometry involves clients blowing air into a machine which produces a graph illustrating normal, restrictive or obstructive airflow. This test will be administered in either primary care or general medical settings as spirometers are generally not available in mental health units. Understanding spirometry constitutes an obvious training need for practitioners.

Differentiating between asthma and COPD is also important so that respiratory distress can be effectively managed. NICE (2004) lists factors for COPD as smoking, rare in people under age 35 and persistent and progressive breathlessness; whereas asthma symptoms are common under age 35, there is variable breathlessness and smoking is a possible factor.

Managing COPD

Our primary role will be screening for COPD which will entail knowledge of signs and symptoms, assessment, diagnosis and management. This will be inter-professional and require liaison with primary care and specialist medical services. Booker (2005) suggests that the aims of treatment for COPD are to

- prevent or ameliorate further disease progression;
- relieve symptoms;
- improve exercise capacity;
- maintain the best possible quality of life;
- prevent exacerbations.

We will play a key role in health education and health promotion from primary prevention, for example, preventing clients from starting smoking; secondary prevention – embarking on behaviour change to support clients in stopping smoking; and tertiary prevention – improving the quality of life of clients with COPD. NICE (2004) outline the key priorities for COPD as

- stop smoking;
- effective inhaled therapy;
- pulmonary rehabilitation for all who need it;
- use non-invasive ventilation;
- manage exacerbations;
- multidisciplinary working.

Care planning will involve inter-professional liaison with a respiratory nurse specialist, a physiotherapist to advise on exercise, and a doctor for advice on specific treatments. As non-specialists our role may be limited to monitoring and evaluation. However, as part of an inter-professional team we would facilitate the day to day management of the treatment plan and report to lead practitioners, most probably a respiratory specialist nurse.

Depending on the severity a care plan will involve:

- medications – inhaler therapy (to include education on proper inhaler technique), oxygen;
- pulmonary rehabilitation;
- dietician – for advice on diet and fluid intake;
- physiotherapy – to advise on exercise;
- social factors – mobility aids for the home, benefits advice for home help or meals on wheels;
- monitoring mental state;
- palliative care.

> **Box 6.4**
> **Exercise**
>
> Which type of evidence based practice guidelines are used as standards for respiratory care in your clinical practice area?

Cough

A cough can be irritating on a continuum of mild, moderate to severe. It is a cardinal symptom of respiratory disorders such as cancer, chest infection or TB. It also occurs in cardiovascular conditions, allergies or the presence of a foreign body obstructing the respiratory tract. Morice *et al.* (2006) define cough in two ways.

- Acute cough: lasting less than 3 weeks, commonly associated with viral upper respiratory tract infection and in the absence of significant co-morbidity, is normally benign and self-limiting. If acute cough presents with any of the following – haemoptysis, breathlessness, fever, chest pain or weight loss, then a chest X-ray is recommended.
- Chronic cough: lasting more than 8 weeks, where most patients present with a dry or minimally productive cough, decrease in quality of life and the presence of significant sputum production, usually indicates primary lung pathology.

The most common cause of cough is irritation, with smoking the most likely provoking agent. However, cough can also be present in COPD and asthma. The longer someone smokes the more persistent the cough will become. Smoking will also leave the person vulnerable to opportunistic lung infections as it decreases the body's defence mechanisms.

Cough assessment

As a baseline measurement ask the client to self-assess cough severity, e.g. on a scale of one (slight cough), to five (severe cough, breathlessness and sputum production). Assessment of cough will involve palpation – sounding the chest and listening for abnormal sounds. Specific questions will address

- Onset – when did it occur, was it sudden or gradual?
- Timing – is it worse at any particular time, e.g. in the morning?
- Duration – are coughing fits long?
- Provocation – what provokes the cough?
- Alleviation – what makes it better?

Other aspects of assessment include the following:

- Does the cough cause chest pain? – inspect chest for signs of trauma or throat for signs of a foreign body
- Is there a history of respiratory illness or cough?
- Have treatments been tried – what, how effective was it?
- Is there sputum production – is blood or odour present?
- Sputum and blood samples may be sent for pathology analysis.

You should also be aware of the client's medical history and whether they are taking any medications that may cause cough, e.g. ACE inhibitors. Indeed some atypical drugs can have adverse effects on the respiratory system, e.g. collapse, respiratory arrest, coughing, pneumonia/pneumonia like symptoms and wheezing in clozapine (Novartis 2008), fatigue, rhinitis, upper respiratory tract infection, coughing in Risperdal (Janssen Pharmaceuticals 2008).

Sputum assessment

If sputum is produced it is important to examine it for signs of blood or odour. This may seem unpleasant but if blood is present it may represent a medical emergency. If a sputum sample is sent to pathology it should be secure, observing infection control and clinical hazard measures. Appropriate containers, packaging and labelling should always be used. Table 6.5 illustrates possible observations from a sputum sample.

Treating cough

Preventing cough by stopping smoking is the first step as this will improve respiratory function and reduce risk of respiratory disorders. Clients may still be at risk of respiratory disorders due to their smoking history but the severity may be reduced. If cough is caused by an infection then treatment of the infection is the priority, ensuring all antibiotic therapies are completed, even when the cough and infection recede. It is important to find out if the client is self-medicating with over the counter cough remedies as these can cause drowsiness. When taken in conjunction with psychotropic drugs drowsiness may be exacerbated.

The client should be advised to rest as much as possible, using extra pillows when in bed and cushions for support when sitting. However, they should also be encouraged to be independent and do some light walking. Homeopathic remedies for cough may also be an option. Menthol vapours or burning incense may help to soothe the airways and clear blocked nasal passages. Folk remedies may also be used by clients, for example, in Ireland a knob of butter on the bridge of the nose is used to ease congestion.

Tuberculosis

Tuberculosis (TB) is a bacterial infection that affects the lungs gradually destroying tissue (Hairon 2007). It is caused by the bacillus *Mycobacterium tuberculosis* and is characterized by the formation of nodular lesions in the tissue (McFerran 2008). TB is a contagious disease spread through spores discharged by someone who has active TB when they cough or sneeze.

In the UK in 2007 the Health Protection Agency (HPA 2008) reported 8,417 confirmed cases of TB, a rate of 13.8 per 100,000 population. London accounted for the largest proportion (39 per cent of UK cases) and the highest regional rate – 43.2 per 100,000. TB now largely affects population subgroups such as ethnic minorities, non-UK born individuals, the homeless, problem drug users and deprived communities. The latter statistic is important for us as our client group is over-represented in such backgrounds. Little is known about the prevalence of TB in our clients. However, two American studies report high prevalence rates in people with SMI in New York;

Table 6.5 Sputum assessment

Sputum type	Possible cause
Pink/frothy	Pulmonary oedema
Yellow/green	Infections
Rusty	Pneumococcal pneumonia
Foul tasting (client report)/ smelling	Anaerobic infection
Viscous	Asthma/infections
Large volumes	Bronchiectasis
Blood stained	Lung cancer, trauma, TB

17 per cent in a population of 71 clients in a day programme (McQuistion *et al.* 1997) and 20 per cent in a sample of 655 individuals admitted to a state psychiatric hospital (Pirl *et al.* 2005).

The symptoms of TB

Individuals with active TB may present with

- Fever
- Night sweats
- Weight loss
- Cough
- Haemoptysis

(Mc Ferran 2008)

Diagnosing active respiratory TB

In the UK, NICE (2006b) includes the following in diagnosing active TB:

- A posterior–anterior chest X-ray should be taken; chest X-ray appearances suggestive of TB should lead to further diagnostic investigation.
- Multiple sputum samples (at least three, with one early morning sample) should be sent for TB microscopy and culture for suspected respiratory TB before starting treatment if possible or, failing that, within 7 days of starting.
- Spontaneously produced sputum should be obtained if possible; otherwise induction of sputum or bronchoscopy and lavage should be used.
- If there are clinical signs and symptoms consistent with a diagnosis of TB, treatment should be started without waiting for culture results.

Management of active TB

A medical model of management is the most appropriate for active TB. NICE (2006b) recommends a 6-month, four-drug initial regimen (6 months of isoniazid and rifampicin supplemented in the first 2 months with pyrazinamide and ethambutol). Compliance is a significant problem with drug treatment for TB. Therefore our primary role will be ensuring compliance and monitoring the course of illness. TB presents a grave threat to public health and we cannot let assumptions about patient autonomy and choice cloud our work here.

The UK has a strict public health law for communicable diseases. Coker *et al.* (2007) examined legal and compulsory measures for TB in Europe. While compulsory treatment for active TB is not practised in the UK, they found compulsory screening, compulsory examination, compulsory detention and exclusion from certain activities for people who are TB active. While the risk is clear it does not diminish the difficulty that ensuring compliance presents. It may not be easy especially for practitioners working with socially excluded groups. The challenges of engagement, developing trust and genuineness are clear. The continual surveillance of clients to ensure compliance, e.g. counting pills or even urine drug screens, can be very threatening and lead to disengagement, the opposite of what is required.

However, as skilled communicators we can effectively convey the necessity of treatment. We should aim to involve clients in treatment and empower them as much as possible through education, providing appropriate information and exploring the possibility of peer support. We need to explain the necessity for continual contact as ensuring their physical well-being and as a means of health education and promoting health.

Another important consideration is your own health and well-being. It is very important that you are up to date will all your immunizations and in this case it is the BCG vaccination.

Asthma

Asthma is an inflammatory disease of the airways associated with episodes of reversible over-reactivity of the airway smooth muscle (Waugh and Grant 2006). During an asthma attack the airways become narrow, restricting oxygen intake. Asthma attacks can be mild or very severe, where breathlessness leads to hypoxia.

Symptoms of asthma

The British Thoracic Society (2008) suggest that features suggestive of asthma in adults are as follows:

- More than one of the following symptoms: wheeze, breathlessness, chest tightness and cough, particularly if:
- symptoms worse at night and in the early morning
- symptoms in response to exercise, allergen exposure and cold air
- symptoms after taking aspirin or beta blockers

Treatment of asthma

Non-pharmacological measures: The environment plays a role in provoking an asthma attack. Clients should avoid exposure to irritants, e.g. dusty and smoky environments. Pollution from traffic may also be a potential problem so clients who live near main roads should keep windows closed as a precaution. Exposure to other irritants needs to be reduced, for example, if the environment is being decorated, then paint fumes may trigger an attack. Good ventilation and avoidance will reduce the likelihood of an attack.

Allergies such as hay fever might cause problems. An adjunct treatment may be required plus minimizing exposure to pollen. The client should be encouraged to find out what the pollen count is so that they can take precautions such as wearing sunglasses and head scarves or baseball caps to prevent pollen resting in their hair.

Pharmacological measures: Compliance with prescribed treatments can prevent an asthma attack or reduce its severity. Clients should be empowered to self-monitor using daily peak flow measurements to record lung function for treatment evaluation. Medications used in asthma can be administered via a number of routes including intravenously, orally but most often by inhalation. They include:

- *Relievers*: Relievers are taken immediately to relieve asthma symptoms by quickly relaxing the muscles surrounding the narrowed airways allowing these to open, making it easier to breathe again (Asthma UK 2004). Examples of relievers include short-acting bronchodilators such as salbutamol and long-acting bronchodilators such as salmeterol, which keeps airways open for a few hours.
- *Preventers*: Preventers control the swelling and inflammation in the airways, stopping them from being sensitive and reducing the risk of severe attacks (Asthma UK 2004). People who require these will also have a reliever prescribed. Examples of preventers include corticosteroid inhalers such as beclomethasone.
- *Corticosteroids tablets*: Corticosteroids are effective in asthma management as they reduce airway inflammation, oedema and secretion of mucus into the airway (BNF 2007). These drugs are used where inhaler therapies have been ineffective. Examples of steroid tablets include dexamethasone and prednisolone.
- *Nebuliser*: In cases of severe asthma attack a nebuliser will be required to administer medicine. A nebuliser is a small plastic container filled with medicine that is attached to a

compressor which blows air into the medicine turning it into a fine mist which is then inhaled via a face mask or mouth-piece (Asthma UK 2004). Medications used in nebuliser medicines are short acting bronchodilators and ipratropium bromide.

Box 6.5
Exercise   List the adverse reactions of salbutamol, prednisolone and beclomethasone.

Management of asthma

People with asthma and co-morbid psychiatric disorders are reported to have poorer asthma control and higher healthcare utilization (Adams *et al.* 2004). Initially we may have to administer medicines until there are improvements in mental state. However, our goal should be empowering clients to be self-medicating by returning inhalers to them when in hospital. This will promote independence and give clients a sense of control over the asthma.

The British Thoracic Society (2008) state that control of asthma is defined as:

- no daytime symptoms;
- no night time awakening due to asthma;
- no need for rescue medication;
- no exacerbations;
- no limitations on activity including exercise;
- normal lung function (in practical terms FEV1 and/or PEF >80 per cent predicted or best) with minimal side effects.

An important aspect of asthma management is inhaler technique. Clients may comply with inhaler therapy but if their technique is faulty they may not be getting optimal doses which can contribute to poor asthma management. Giraud and Roche (2002) found that poor inhaler technique, mainly due to poor coordination, was associated with poor asthma control. They suggest that education of clients in good inhaler technique is an important factor in effectively managing asthma. Another method of ensuring optimal dosing is using spacers as these help to deliver asthma medicine to the lungs, making the inhaler easier to use (Asthma UK 2004).

Pneumonia

Pneumonia is a lower respiratory tract infection and is defined as inflammation of the lung caused by bacteria, in which the alveoli become filled with inflammatory cells and the lung becomes solid (McFerran 2008). Watson (2008a) suggests that pneumonia can be classified in two types – the site of infection, e.g. bronchial pneumonia; or if it is caused by an organism as in bacterial pneumonia.

Pathophysiology

When the alveoli contain fluid this takes up space, reducing the amount of oxygen that can enter into the lungs causing inadequate gaseous exchange. This reduces the levels of oxygen in the blood which leads to breathlessness, discomfort and tachypnoea. In someone who is frail or has other risk factors for respiratory ill health, it can be very severe and lead to hypoxia. Therefore pneumonia can be a life threatening condition in people who are physically ill or frail. The risk factors for pneumonia are as follows (Watson 2008a):

- Pre-existing illness such as
  - Renal impairment
  - Diabetes
  - COPD
  - Asthma
- People who are immuno-compromised, e.g. HIV positive, transplant patients, very young or intubated
- History of alcohol or substance misuse
- Poor nutritional health

Diagnosing pneumonia

Hoare and Lim (2006) outline the signs and symptoms of pneumonia as

- shortness of breath
- pleuritic chest pain
- cough
- production of sputum
- rigors or night sweats
- confusion
- raised respiratory rate
- fever of $> 38°C$
- focal chest signs: decreased chest expansion, dullness on percussion, decreased entry of air, bronchial breathing, and crackles (none, some, or all of these may be present).

Other types of diagnostic tests will be needed to confirm pneumonia. Blood tests that examine full blood count especially for white blood cells will identify any infection. Samples can be taken to investigate if cultures are present in sputum. These will identify organisms for which appropriate treatment can be given.

Treatment

The treatment plan is likely to be inter-professional and your role may be as a co-facilitator and liaison with the other practitioners involved. The first stage of treatment would aim to promote oxygen intake into the blood stream in order to manage breathlessness and any hypoxia. Regular recording and documentation of physical observations is important.

Medication may be required in two forms: pain relief for any chest pain during respiration and antibiotics to fight any infection. Antibiotics should be safely administered until the course has been completed. Physiotherapists may be required to provide advice on posture and the expectoration of sputum. They may have to provide chest massage which will help the client to cough up and expel sputum.

Depending on severity the client may be on bed rest. This presents risks that require management, for example:

- Hydration: reduce the risk of dehydration by ensuring adequate fluid balance as the person may be dependent on staff to bring fluids.
- Appetite: liquid nutritional substitutes may be prescribed until the pneumonia recedes and appetite returns.
- Posture: encourage upright posture to prevent aspiration when eating and drinking.
- Skin: encourage the client to refrain from lying and sitting continually to reduce risk of pressure sores. Light mobility may be required.

Respiratory assessment

The primary purpose of respiratory assessment is to determine the adequacy of gaseous exchange (Moore 2007). Physical assessment skills required for respiratory assessment include observation, inspection, palpation and auscultation. Ferns and Chojnacka (2006) suggest that clinical assessment and physical assessment skills are the dominant variables in respiratory assessment. Practical considerations for privacy, dignity and respect also apply here as disrobing will be required.

The first stage of respiratory assessment is observation. By looking and listening to someone we can get a crude assessment of their respiratory health. The process of ventilation should be smooth and noiseless. On hearing abnormal sounds we should assume there is a problem. This is important as observation will determine whether the assessment is of an emergency or routine nature. Obvious respiratory distress should be treated as a medical emergency. Observation will also prompt us to ask closed questions if open questions lead to breathlessness.

Breathlessness

Breathlessness is a common complaint in respiratory conditions and something that needs considering during assessment. The Medical Research Council dyspnoea scale offers a guide to assessing the severity of breathlessness. It has five levels of breathlessness ranging from 1 – not troubled by breathlessness except on strenuous exercise – to 5 – too breathless to leave the house, or breathless when dressing or undressing (see NICE 2004: 9).

Visual observation

- Skin colour, peripheral cyanosis, nicotine stains on hair/fingers;
- Respiratory effort when answering questions (repeated stoppages for breaths, unable to complete a long sentence);
- Posture during breathing effort bent over or very erect;
- Effort when breathing (Is the client using accessory muscles to help breathing? Observe clavicles and neck for movement);
- Expressions of pain or discomfort;
- Is chest movement symmetrical? (Does chest expand and contract in unison?);
- Is there breathlessness on minor exertion?
- Finger clubbing is a symptom of respiratory illness. Here the tips of the fingers appear swollen and on palpation are spongy.

Auditory observation

Listen for abnormal breathing sounds:

- Cough;
- Crackles (high-pitched, popping sounds heard during inspiration due to delay in airways reopening);
- Wheezes (whistling sounds caused by narrow airways, e.g. obstruction caused by a foreign object or mucous secretions);

- Rhonchi (an abnormal musical noise produced by air passing through narrowed bronchi, McFerran 2008);
- Stridor (noise heard on inspiration due to trachea or larynx obstruction, McFerran 2008).

Inspection

Examination of the chest during ventilation:

- Equal and symmetrical lung expansion on inspiration;
- Chest shape, e.g. barrel chest due to COPD;
- Observe the skin for any scarring or trauma;
- Inspect the fingers for evidence of finger clubbing.

Palpation

- Is the trachea in its usual position? Deviation of the trachea may occur following asphyxiation trauma.
- Can you feel lymph nodes on the neck?
- Gently trace over the rib cage for evidence of swelling or tenderness.

Auscultation and percussion

Auscultation involves using a stethoscope to assess breathing sounds, while percussion is tapping the thoracic area to identify foreign sounds. Percussion and auscultation may be performed by the doctor. However, these are the types of skills that nurses should be acquiring in order to extend practice. Further questions that can be used to structure the assessment include:

- Is there any pain?
- Is there a family history of respiratory disorders?
- What is the client's smoking history?: current and past history (calculate pack years[1]); history of attempts to quit; have there been any changes in smoking habit?
- What is the client's occupational history (to determine work related exposure to irritants)?
- What provokes or reduces breathlessness?
- Has there been recent weight loss?
- Is the client waking from sleep at night due to breathlessness (possible orthopnoea)?
- Does breathlessness cause mobility problems?
- Has the client had the flu or pneumococcal vaccinations?

Clinical observations

Respiratory assessment is more than counting the rate of respirations. Other observations include the following (see also Chapter 3):

- respiratory rate between 12 and 18, regular, effortless, no foreign sounds
- pulse oximetry of 95 per cent or above
- PEFR measurement

---

1 Prignot (1987) defines a pack year smoked as 1 packet of cigarettes or 20g of tobacco smoked each day for a full year (one cigarette is equal to one gram).

- central cyanosis (look under client's tongue for blueness)
- temperature (to determine fever)
- full blood count (is breathlessness related to anaemia or chest infection?)
- arterial blood gases (assesses client's respiratory and metabolic status e.g. acidosis)
- spirometry
- chest X-ray
- sputum sample

Emergency respiratory assessment

Emergency respiratory assessment will be required when we find someone in a state of collapse or with acute breathlessness. Key aspects of an emergency respiratory assessment include:

- is the client too breathless to speak?
- tachycardia, i.e. a pulse rate over 110 beats per minute in adults
- bradycardia, i.e. a pulse rate under 50 beats per minute in adults
- tachypnoea, i.e. a respiratory rate of 25 breaths or more per minute in adults
- bradypnoea, i.e. a respiratory rate under 10 breaths or more per minute in adults
- cyanosis: peripheral (fingers or lips) and central (under the tongue)
- O_2 saturation less than 90 per cent
- central/left sided chest pain with nausea (possible neck or jaw pain also)
- altered consciousness level – confusion or drowsiness
- is it hyperventilation due to anxiety?

Smoking cessation

Smoking is a modifiable risk factor and a key health promotion intervention is smoking cessation. This includes education about the negative effects of smoking and the positive benefits of giving up. With support and smoking cessation aids, smoking behaviour can be reduced and stopped. If clients do not accept this advice that is unfortunate; we cannot give nicotine replacement compulsorily. However, we must continue to offer advice and empower them to change this risk behaviour in a supportive way.

One approach to broaching the subject of smoking cessation is the 'five As' approach (Raw et al. 1998):

- Ask about smoking.
- Advise people to stop.
- Assess motivation to stop and the need for pharmacotherapy.
- Assist with prescription or referral to behavioural support.
- Arrange follow up.

Indeed NICE (2006b) recommend that brief smoking cessation interventions should include, among other things, advising clients to stop smoking and referring them to smoking cessation services. Practitioners should be able to give smoking cessation/stop smoking support contacts; in the UK this would be telephone numbers for the NHS Stop Smoking Services.

There are three main aspects of smoking cessation that are used separately or in conjunction with each other:

- counselling support;
- prescription of medication, e.g. bupropion hydrochloride;
- nicotine replacement therapy, e.g. patches.

The first stage of the process should be an assessment of smoking:

- type of tobacco consumption – cigarettes, hand rolling tobacco, pipe;
- number/quantity of cigarettes, tobacco used per day;
- any particular rituals observed, e.g. a cigarette and a cup of tea;
- any factors that induce smoking, e.g. anxiety, stress;
- any factors that reduce the need to smoke.

The second stage is assessing client's motivation to stop smoking with questions such as

- Do you want to stop smoking for good?
- Are you interested in making a serious attempt to stop in the near future?
- Are you interested in receiving help with your cessation attempt?

(West 2004)

These questions can be phrased so as to rate our client's motivation using simple scales. For example:
On a scale of 1 (not at all) to 5 (very much so):

- How strong is your desire to stop smoking for good?
- How interested are you in making a serious attempt to stop in the near future?
- How interested are you interested in receiving help with your cessation attempt?

A smoking cessation group might benefit clients in offering peer support and encouragement. This approach will also be beneficial in effectively managing practitioner's time. However, individual support should also be offered, e.g. through telephone support and follow up. Group support may involve the following:

- Outline the reasons for smoking.
- Outline the reasons for stopping (emphasize these).
- Explore factors that make quitting difficult.
- Plan to reduce or eliminate these factors.
- Help with setting realistic goals.
- Develop coping skills without nicotine.
- Provide a physical health check.
- Provide general health education advice.

Nicotine replacement therapy (NRT) – gum, patches or inhalers – should be used in the short term to support with the nicotine withdrawal. Smoking should have stopped before initiating NRT (BNF 2007). Medication may also be considered for very heavy smokers. Bupropion hydrochloride, once used as an antidepressant, is often used in smoking cessation, although its mode of action is not clear (BNF 2007). If this is prescribed then we should be aware of any adverse reactions and contra-indications. Finally, smoking cessation should not only be an issue for clients; if you smoke maybe you could avail of this also?

How effective is smoking cessation?

One problem with smoking cessation is the rate of relapses once support has finished. Some people have repeated relapses before stopping and some people cannot stop at all. Raw *et al.* (2005) summarize the evidence around smoking cessation as this:

- Nicotine replacement helps smokers unwilling or unable to stop achieve sustained reduction in cigarette consumption.
- This reduction is accompanied by a reduction in smoke intake.
- Smoking reduction using NRT increases motivation to stop smoking.

- Smoking reduction using NRT increases subsequent cessation.

Practitioners should encourage and support clients to stop smoking. We should reiterate the positive benefits of stopping and get clients to focus on these rather than dwell on relapse. This is very important for clients that have respiratory conditions and smoke. Clients self-reporting of positive health gains should be used as further examples for motivation, increasing confidence and self-esteem. We should offer practical solutions when cravings arise. This will include

- educating clients that cravings will arise and can be unpleasant;
- preparing clients for cravings, e.g. draw on past experience;
- educating clients that cravings can be overcome without recourse to smoking. For example, suggesting clients chew a piece of gum or do something that will divert their thoughts;
- emphasizing the positive aspects of stopping. Should relapse occur then this should be acknowledged but the emphasis remains on accentuating the positive.

Box 6.7   How do you refer someone for smoking cessation?
Exercise

Smoking cessation: the challenges and rewards

The addictive nature of nicotine and subsequent unpleasantness of withdrawal can be a barrier to quitting. The added anxiety and stress of trying to cope without smoking may be a further deterrent. However, clients are often excluded from health promotion services so they may also face exclusion from smoking cessation services. Frequent relapses may be de-motivating and engender feelings of powerlessness. When individuals become dispirited this may decrease their motivation to quit. This may reinforce the fatalist attitudes of practitioners or weaken the resolve of staff that are motivated to implement smoking cessation.

Wild and Byrne (2006) suggest that the relationship between smoking and obesity is complex: smoking is associated with lower BMI whereas smoking cessation is linked with weight gain. Therefore a holistic lifestyle approach is important and should include diet and physical activity advice in conjunction with smoking cessation.

Mental health units have been described as un-therapeutic (Samarasekera 2007), therefore providing a structured and meaningful day can be difficult. This is where physical health takes on a whole organization approach rather than an individual client nurse interaction. If clients are motivated to stop smoking services should respond creatively. Banning smoking from premises is an approach, but it is flawed as people can smoke outside. Providing a structured day with various diversional activities, support groups, healthy lifestyles groups, exercise groups, for example, a walking group are some ways that might help. But these are difficult to institute without creativity and resources – not only financial but also in respect to staff skills.

The rewards for stopping smoking are evident. These can be split into health related gains and financial gains. The health related gains include a reduced risk of worse health although some damage may have already been done by the previous smoking history. We can calculate very crude financial costs of smoking. The UK prevalence of schizophrenia is 1 in 100 people (Royal College of Psychiatrists 2007). The UK adult population of 18–60 years is 46,000,000 (ONS 2005). The number of people with schizophrenia in this group is 460,000 (46,000,000 / 100 = 460,000). Estimates suggest smoking rates of 80 per cent in this group (McNeill 2001) (80 per cent of 460,000 = 368,000 people). If each person smoked 20 cigarettes a day, at £4 pounds per packet, this amounts to (368,000 × £4) = £1,472,000 per day, £10,304,000 per week or £537,280,000 per year. UK duty on a pack of twenty cigarettes is 22 per cent of the retail price (HM Revenue and Customs, no date). Therefore clients who smoke contribute around £118,201,600 in UK tax (22 per cent of £537,280,000).

Care planning

Using Roper, Logan and Tierney's (1996) model of Activities of Daily Living, we can devise and structure a care plan for someone with a respiratory condition. The care plan will aim to restore normal functioning, or as close as possible. However, with physical conditions and the complex interaction of a matrix of factors, it is prudent to have an emergency contingency care plan.

Again our role in care planning will depend on the severity of the presentation but we will be in a position to screen for respiratory disorders and collaborate in an inter-professional care plan. Here our role will be facilitating clinical observations, recording, documenting and communicating these to the team and liaising with the medical or specialist respiratory nurse practitioner. As there is a co-morbid presence of anxiety and depression with respiratory disorders, our role here will be as primary carers, looking after the mental and emotional health of our clients.

Treating and managing respiratory illness

Clinical priorities include

- normalizing respiration rate;
- ensuring adequate oxygenation of the blood and tissues;
- preventing hypoxia;
- correcting the cause of/reducing the impact of respiratory disorders;
- ensuring compliance with treatment;
- continual monitoring;
- smoking cessation using NRT.

Table 6.6 provides an illustration of factors that you might consider when writing a care plan for someone suffering from a respiratory problem using Roper, Logan and Tierney's Model (1996).

Summary of key points

High smoking prevalence in mental health means a greater risk of more respiratory (and cardio-vascular) disorders in our client group. Respiratory assessment is an important part of our work and we should be able to conduct a safe and thorough examination. A medical approach will be one aspect of the assessment but nurses should follow this up with a psycho-social assessment. The British Thoracic Society (2006) state that 44 per cent of all deaths from respiratory disease are associated with social class inequalities. This presents a clear public health challenge to us as our clients come from this high risk social group. Therefore assessment would also explore smoking behaviour and attitudes to stopping, living conditions and supportive environments.

As health promoters we must also remember that one in eight of all lung cancer cases are among people who have never touched a cigarette (UK Lung Cancer coalition 2005). In the debate about the rights of smokers to smoke we should remember that non-smokers are put at risk of developing respiratory disorders due to passive smoking.

We need to increase our knowledge of pharmacology as a necessary by-product of the prevalence of physical illness in our clients. Greater awareness of adverse drug reactions associated with treating respiratory conditions is needed. Practitioners should have appropriate training

Table 6.6 An illustration of factors that you might consider when writing a care plan for someone suffering from a respiratory problem

Activity of daily living	Example of care planning activity
1 Maintaining a safe environment	This might relate to homeostasis as the internal body environment. Our aim is to restore normal respiration rate or as close as can be, given any respiratory tract damage. We also want to prevent/reduce the risk of hypoxia. We can achieve this through • monitoring baseline observations • monitoring physical interventions such as medications • evaluating the effectiveness of treatment • prescription of oxygen therapy • appropriate immunizations offered as a primary prevention of respiratory infections • re-visiting care plan if condition deteriorates. Physical environment is also important as it is important to limit the amount of physical exertion required when moving around. The home environment may need to be adapted to minimize the levels of exertion, e.g. installation of stair lift or other mobility aids, adapting showers, installing hand rails and other supports.
2 Breathing	Monitoring respirations is a core observation. With respiratory problems breathlessness is a clinical feature. Breathlessness can be anxiety provoking due to the associated discomfort and its role as a reinforcing agent of illness. Breathing should also be monitored when the client is asleep. Observations and interventions include: • respiration rate • presence of cyanosis • pulse oximetry • oxygen therapy • posture when sitting or lying • arterial blood gases • review of antipsychotic medications • involvement of physiotherapy for advice on exercise or removing excess sputum • collecting sputum samples for pathology and assessing any cough
3 Communicating	Care planning and treatment for respiratory problems can be very complex. Any instructions or explanations should • be jargon free • be easy to understand • seek regular feedback to ensure comprehension • seek clarification that things have been understood. You should also reassure the client to alleviate any anxiety. Encourage them to express feelings and develop psychological coping strategies, or acceptance of a physical illness. This will decrease anxiety as they find they can still have a social life as long as they are not overexerting. You should also try to establish if there are any peer support groups that they or their carers/family can attend in the community.
4 Mobilizing	While encouraging fitness is important this should not be too strenuous. Set small and safe targets, e.g. • involve physiotherapy to develop an exercise plan; • walking short distances gradually increasing this; • encourage rest also and explore the best postures for optimal ventilation; • consider relaxation therapy to help the resting process and cope with stress;

(Continued Overleaf)

Table 6.6 continued

Activity of daily living	Example of care planning activity
	• encourage the use of walking aids. This might feel disempowering for the client but our aim is to promote independence. This should be emphasized to them, if they use aids appropriately they will become more independent. (Also refer to maintaining a safe environment above.)
5 Eating and drinking	Diet may need to change as in respiratory conditions weight gain or weight loss may occur. The dietician can advise on appropriate diets in whichever circumstances but as a general rule diets should be well balanced: • encourage fruit and fibre; • control calories to prevent/increase weight; • explore healthy cooking options/meal choices depending on level of independence; • use of food supplements such as Complan; • promote a low salt diet; • reduce/abstain from alcohol intake. Occupational therapy can help with cooking skills.
6 Eliminating	Levels of physical activity may reduce so it is important to prevent elimination problems such as constipation (as this is also a side effect of antipsychotic medication). • encourage adequate hydration; • introduce dietary changes to promote bowel function; • take bloods to monitor electrolytes.
7 Personal cleansing and dressing	In some cases assistance may be required but the goal should be to promote independence. This will illustrate to the client that they can still function normally. • ensure safety when bathing/showering as this can be tiring; • use shower seat aids to minimize exertion; • observe skin integrity – reduced oxygenation of blood may compromise skin integrity; • show respect for privacy and dignity.
8 Maintaining body temperature	Temperature should be monitored regularly if the respiratory condition is caused by an infection. If medication is given e.g. paracetamol, temperature should be monitored to evaluate the effectiveness of this. • treat any infection; • ensure adequate hydration; • use a fan or cool flannel to reduce temperature.
9 Working and playing	Refer to mobilizing above. • time off work may be required for those who are employed; • ensuring appropriate benefits are in situ, e.g. if homes have to be renovated to help mobility; • recreational activities may have to be less strenuous initially; • explore local self-help or support groups that might have social activities.
10 Sleeping	Sleep may be affected by breathing problems. We should observe for sleep difficulties and consider commencing a sleep chart. • use of extra pillows to assist breathing; • discourage sleeping during the day; • consider medication if required.

11 Expressing sexuality	Depending on the severity of the problem
	• sexual activity may decrease initially due to respiratory condition;
	• explain this to the client and partner to promote understanding;
	• reassure that sexual activity will return but this will take some time.
12 Dying	Clients may be preoccupied with death or dying
	• allow clients to express fears;
	• reassure that with treatment and lifestyle changes life can still be enjoyed;
	• discuss fears of the future openly and discourage catastrophic thinking;
	• encourage joining a support group to get peer support;
	• palliative care may need to be considered depending on the severity and associated outcomes. Clients at this stage should be empowered to plan their death so that they retain control of their life. Advanced directives may be required so we may have to seek legal advice and advocate for the client's rights with this.

and clinical instruments required to conduct a respiratory assessment. It is through screening and identifying signs and symptoms of respiratory disorders that we can promote the physical health of our clients. Thus a more appropriate exchange should be:

Q: Do your clients cough?
A: Yes, they cough all the time because they may have a smoking related respiratory disorder.

Quick quiz

1 What is external respiration?
2 What is internal respiration?
3 Define diffusion.
4 Describe the effects of smoking on the respiratory system.
5 What is the role of the mental health nurse in respiratory health?

7 Assessing nutrition, diet and physical activity

By the end of this chapter you will have:

- Explored the importance of nutrition, diet and physical activity
- Examined the prevalence of obesity and diabetes in our client group
- Explored physical activity in clients
- Defined obesity and examined risk factors
- Examined metabolic syndrome and its management in clients
- Examined screening for metabolic conditions

Box 7.1
Exercise
What is the prevalence of overweight and obesity in your client group?

Introduction

Nutrition is an input to, and foundation for, health and development (WHO 2008b). However, there are great concerns about the nutritional health of populations. Whether food scares or the obesity epidemic, diet, nutrition and physical inactivity are never far from the health or general media. Evidence suggests that excessive consumption of energy-rich foods, e.g. processed foods, drinks containing saturated and transfats, sugars and salt, encourages weight gain (WHO 2003).

Table 7.1 illustrates the prevalence of obesity measured using the body mass index (BMI) scale. In respect to the UK general population we know that most adults in England are overweight; obesity causes 30,000 deaths a year and shortens life by 9 years on average (Select

Table 7.1 The prevalence of obesity measured using the body mass index (BMI) scale

	Prevalence of obesity	
	Male %	**Female %**
USA[1]	33.3	35.3
Australia[2]	17.8	15.1
European[3]	10–27	up to 38
UK[4]	24	24

Sources: 1 the National Center for Health Statistics (2007); 2 Australian Institute of Health and Welfare (2006); 3 Lobstein *et al.* (2005); 4 Craig and Shelton 2008

Committee on Public Accounts 2002); the prevalence of diabetes is 3.6 per cent, around 2.3 million people (Diabetes UK 2007); physical activity levels are low. In 2004, 35 per cent of men and 24 per cent of women met government recommendations for physical activity (The Information Centre 2006). If we look at our clients as a general population sub-group we see a worsening picture that warrants special investigation. Research on diet, obesity and physical activity in mental health shows the following:

- Lifestyle factors that cause obesity, such as low levels of exercise and poor diet are present in people with mental illness (Brown *et al.* 1999).
- Kendrick (1996) found that of 101 people with SMI living in the community 26 were clinically obese.
- McCreadie *et al.* (1998) found that people with schizophrenia made poor dietary choices characterized by a high fat, low fibre dietary intake.
- Daumit *et al.* (2005) in a survey of outpatients at two psychiatric centres in the USA found they were less physically active than the general population and those who were more inactive had fewer social contacts.

Reasons for high prevalence in people with mental illness

The main cause of poor nutrition, diet and lack of physical activity in our clients is that they are part of a general population that has the same problems. In this regard our clients are quite 'normal'. However, our clients, coming from a lower social class, are more exposed to lifestyle risk factors as inequalities in health affect them disproportionately (see Chapter 1). They live in more deprived areas, face increased social exclusion and unemployment and lack material wealth.

Clinical factors affecting diet and physical activity are very complex and include adverse drug reactions that provoke weight gain, metabolic disorders and induce movement disorders that may make performing exercise difficult. Negative symptoms of psychotic illnesses may inhibit motivation to engage in lifestyle programmes, while negative staff attitudes regarding these constitute a further barrier to change. Our client group is also socially excluded and may not be able to access health promotion and health education services as the general population do.

The result of this is that our clients have an increased risk of higher mortality and morbidity. Why? The debate is essentially balanced on poor lifestyle choices and adverse drug reactions. This chapter will explore the impact of poor lifestyle choices on clients' physical health. It will commence with a recap of basic nutrition and move onto obesity, physical activity and diet and nutrition. It will examine nutritional assessment and fluid balance before exploring diabetes and metabolic syndrome. It will finish by exploring care planning for diet, nutrition and obesity.

**Box 7.2
Exercise**   What is the recommended daily calorie intake for (a) men and (b) women?

Nutrients and nutrition

Micronutrients enable the body to produce enzymes, hormones and other substances essential for proper growth and development (WHO 2008c). Nutrients include carbohydrates, proteins, vitamins, fats and minerals. An overabundance or an inadequate supply can cause physical illness. The following outlines the main nutrient groups involved in a balanced diet.

Carbohydrates

Carbohydrates can be split into two main groups:

- Simple carbohydrates – sugars
- Complex carbohydrates – starch

Carbohydrates are essential as an energy source. Carbohydrates are found in bread, potatoes, pasta, rice and cereals, as these are generally high in starch. Carbohydrates make us feel full and as they release energy slowly they avoid sudden drops in blood glucose that result in hunger pangs.

Proteins

Proteins are composed of amino-acids and are crucial for muscle, tissue and organ growth and development. There are two main groups of amino-acids:

- Nonessential amino-acids – these can be manufactured by the body.
- Essential amino-acids – these cannot be manufactured by the body so need to be taken in our diet.

Proteins are found in meat, fish, eggs, dairy products and pulses such as lentils and chick-peas.

Fats

There are various types of fats:

- Saturated fats – found in animal fat
- Unsaturated fats – these come in two forms; mono-saturated fats found in olives, and poly-unsaturated fats found in nuts and seeds
- Triglycerides – fats found in meat, dairy products and cooking oils

Cholesterol is produced by the body and ingested in our diet. It is found in milk, eggs and meat. Cholesterol is an important risk factor in the development of heart disease. There are two key types that it is important for practitioners to know about:

- High density lipoproteins (HDLs) are made up of protein and a small amount of fat.
- Low density lipoproteins (LDLs) are made up of fat and a small amount of proteins.

(Krozier *et al.* 2008)

HDLs contain less fat and are referred to as 'good' cholesterol. LDLs, containing more fat, are known as 'bad' cholesterol. The National Cholesterol Education Program (NCEP) (2002) in the USA states the causes of low HDL cholesterol include

- elevated serum triglycerides
- overweight and obesity
- physical inactivity
- cigarette smoking
- very high carbohydrate intakes (>60 percent of total energy intake)
- T2D
- certain drugs (beta-blockers, anabolic steroids, progestational agents)
- genetic factors

Omega-3 fatty acids

Omega-3 cannot be manufactured by the body so we take it in our diet or through nutritional supplements. Oily fish such as salmon and tuna contain Omega-3 which is rich in docosa-hexaenoic acid (DHA) and eicosapentaenoic acid (EPA); DHA and EPA are key components of our eyes and brain (Ruxton 2004).

Omega-3 has been used to treat a number of physical and mental illnesses. For example, it has been be used to reduce triglyceride levels and may also be used in conjunction with a statin to manage hyperlipidaemia (British National Formulary 2007). Peet (2003) reports on a series of studies that used essential fatty acids such as Omega-3 in the treatment of schizophrenia and depression. Healy *et al.* (2005) also report on the use of Omega-3 as an adjunct in clozapine therapy and offer a summary of evidence of the use of fish oils in schizophrenia (p. 69).

Vitamins and vitamin deficiency

Vitamins are essential components of a healthy diet. Insufficient vitamin intake is associated with a number of physical conditions and sustained vitamin deficiency has serious implications for physical health.

Vitamins come in two main types:

- Fat soluble vitamins can be stored by the body so a daily intake is not really necessary (Kozier *et al.* 2008); examples include vitamins A, D, E and K.
- Water soluble vitamins are vitamins that the body cannot store and thus needs a daily supply (Kozier *et al.* 2008); examples include vitamin C and B-complex vitamins such as B1, B2 and B12.

Fat soluble vitamins

- *Vitamin A* is found in eggs, fish, milk and dairy products. It helps strengthen the immune system and it helps with vision as deficiency causes night-blindness.
- *Vitamin D* is found in eggs, liver and fish; it also synthesizes in the body naturally from sunlight. Vitamin D deficiency can cause rickets, a bone disorder.
- *Vitamin E* is found in oils such as olive oil. It is also found in cereals containing nuts and wholegrain wheat in bread. Vitamin E helps to protect cell membranes by acting as an antioxidant (Food Standards Agency no date). Vitamin E deficiency can lead to neuro-muscular, vascular and reproductive systems problems (Expert Group on Vitamins and Minerals 2003).
- *Vitamin K* is found in green vegetables such as cabbage and broccoli. The body requires vitamin K for effective clotting of the blood and a deficiency results in excessive bleeding.

(Ingham and O'Reilly 2005)

Water soluble vitamins

- *Vitamin B_1*, or thiamin, is found in cereals, vegetables, wholegrain bread and fruit. Thiamin deficiency can cause beriberi which affects the nervous system. Symptoms include lethargy and fatigue. In chronic alcohol abuse a lack of thiamin leads to Wernicke-Korsakoff Syndrome, a form of brain damage (Alcohol Concern 2003). This is normally irreversible.
- *Vitamin B_{12}* is found in meat products, fish and dairy products. Deficiency can lead to anaemia and neurological damage (Ingham and O'Reilly 2005). High levels of alcohol consumption can also lead to vitamin B_{12} deficiency.
- *Vitamin C*, or ascorbic acid, is found in citrus fruits and broccoli. Vitamin C deficiency can

lead to scurvy. Scurvy is characterized by swollen bleeding gums and a rash of tiny bleeding spots around the hair follicles (McFerran 2008).

Minerals

These are nutrients that the body needs to develop and sustain many key functions. Minerals that we require in recommended daily amounts include sodium, potassium, iron and calcium. Minerals play a key role in electrolyte balance, cardiovascular function, bone development and metabolism.

* * *

A healthy diet will entail having a good balance of the nutrients outlined above. However, food preparation is also important. While potatoes may be a good source of carbohydrates, chips will be high in fat content. Food preparation is an important behavioural change and we should be encouraging a move away from eating predominantly fried foods to foods that are grilled or steamed.

Obesity

Obesity is an excess of body fat. Recent news media reports of an obesity epidemic have prompted great fear and debate in wider society and government departments. Obesity and being overweight are serious public health concerns due to their association with increased physical illness and death. Preventing obesity is a key public health aim as it produces a great health gain for the population in respect to decreased mortality and morbidity and an economic gain for health services.

Diseases and conditions associated with obesity include the following (NICE 2006c):

- Sleep apnoea
- Respiratory disease
- Breathlessness
- Asthma
- Social isolation and depression
- Daytime sleepiness and fatigue
- Musculoskeletal problems, e.g. bad back
- Oedema/cellulitis

There are three ways in which we can monitor weight gain and obesity in our client group: (i) BMI, (ii) waist circumference and (iii) waist-hip ratio (see Chapter 3). The target BMI is estimated at 21 to 23 (World Cancer Research Fund 2007). Therefore we could set the target BMI for our clients at the higher end of this estimate (i.e. 23) due to their exposure to adverse drug reactions. While this represents a goal to aim for, our objective should also include integrating healthy eating, increasing physical activity and reducing alcohol consumption and smoking as part of a wider healthier lifestyle strategy.

Using the BMI score is not without controversy. An athlete may have a BMI of 35 but they will not necessarily be obese as their weight is likely to be lean muscle rather than body fat. Dougherty and Lister (2008) also comment that an apparently normal weight may mask muscle wasting. When monitoring weight you might also ask 'clothes fit questions'. For example:

Nurse: Your weight is 15 and a half stones, is that usual?
Abdul: No, I've put on weight recently.

Nurse: What is your normal weight?
Abdul: Around 12 and a half stones.
Nurse: Are the clothes you are wearing now your normal size?
Abdul: No, I've gone up two sizes.
Nurse: What is your usual waist size?
Abdul: 32 inches.
Nurse: What is it now?
Abdul: 36 inches.
Nurse: When were you last your usual weight?
Abdul: About four months ago.

This exchange gives an indication of rapid weight gain. It may also highlight a social problem – does Abdul have enough money to spend on clothes that only fit for a short period of time? What can we do to help him in this respect?

Box 7.3
Exercise
How can we help clients, such as Abdul, with similar social problems that impact on physical health?

Relevance of obesity to mental health

Tackling obesity is an important priority because it is an important public health concern. Weight gain and obesity contribute to cardio-respiratory disorders and are risk factors associated with CHD, hypertension, type 2 diabetes, cancer and high blood cholesterol. Obesity also increases mortality and morbidity in our client group.

Adverse drug reactions are also an important consideration. Weight gain and obesity are linked to many psychotropic drugs (see Chapter 8). This factor makes tackling obesity more complicated where the clinical decision between a client's mental health (psychosis) and physical health (obesity) is a fine balance. Healy (2005) suggests that the cosmetic side effect of weight gain is treated as trivial by practitioners who believe that dopamine-related side effects are more important. This particular debate needs to be had in mental health nursing.

Trying to establish the exact causal link between obesity and our clients may lead clinicians to hold off on interventions until the 'evidence' can be generated. However, our duty of care to clients must include their physical health as well as their mental health. Tackling obesity can produce important mental health benefits such as increasing clients' self-esteem and compliance with medication. It should be adopted as routine clinical practice.

Assessing and managing obesity

Lowe and Lubos (2008), in a review of effectiveness of weight management interventions, paint a disheartening picture. Based on current evidence effectiveness of either psycho-educational interventions or of programmes including educational and exercise components is limited. However, it is not really surprising that little evidence exists, given the neglected state of physical health in general and of exercise as an intervention in particular (Callaghan 2004).

We require systems for identifying risk factors and screening clients for physical conditions. These systems will prioritize primary, secondary and tertiary interventions. A case example for obesity is illustrated below.

Case example: Screening for obesity risk factors

Rationale

Obesity is prevalent in our client group due to lifestyle factors and adverse drug reactions. Reducing obesity is a key government health aim and NICE (2006c) have a clinical guideline on obesity that can guide best practice.

Process

Identify clients at risk:

- Clients with a BMI over 30 or
- Clients may be overweight (BMI 25–29.9) but have other risk factors e.g. T2D, CHD or dyslipidaemia

Risk factors in obesity

The following risk factors should be recorded, along with their status (present, absent or not known):

- dyslipidaemia
- diabetes
- other physical conditions
- family history of diabetes or cardiovascular illness
- current medication
- estimated current calorie intake
- estimated salt intake
- ethnicity
- smoking
- current alcohol intake
- current exercise levels

The risk estimate for complications of obesity should then be calculated as low, moderate or high.

Care planning

Following assessment a care plan is required. This should be realistic, taking into account the realities faced by our clients. It should focus on small, achievable, measurable goals. This provides the client with evidence of achievement which can increase motivation and self-esteem. Care plans should be designed to reduce weight, or in the case of adverse drug reactions, slow down the rate at which weight is gained. Interventions will depend on the severity of obesity or weight gain and any associated complications. The care plan should be clearly documented and reviewed according to local and professional standards.

Aims

- To reduce weight safely and restore a healthy BMI. A maximum weekly weight loss of 0.5–1 kg with an end goal of losing 5–10 per cent of original weight is recommended (NICE 2006c).

- Increase physical activity. A structured, active day will minimize the likelihood of boredom, which might result in snacking. Activity programmes must be safe for clients and include activities they enjoy.
- Change attitudes. Behavioural therapy may help clients to change lifestyles. Changes should be planned and staged rather than 'all or nothing' as non-achievement may reduce motivation.

Implementation

- Health education and promotion around lifestyle, diet and activity
- Referral to a specialist mental health dietician for a weight management plan. General dietary advice will include
  - controlling calorie intake, aiming for around 1,500Kcals per day for women and 2,000Kcals for men. Advice should be sought from a dietician about a calorie controlled diet;
  - increase fruit and fibre intake;
  - decrease in salt intake;
  - decrease saturated fat intake;
  - decrease alcohol and tobacco intake.
- Referral to occupational therapy for advice on food preparation

Increasing physical activity

- Baseline observations should be monitored regularly.
- Introduce gradual and realistic activities as overweight clients may be limited in their physical ability, e.g. introduce light exercise such as brisk walking building up to light jogging.
- Set measurable goals, e.g. begin with 15 minutes walking five times per week and build up from this as stamina increases. Measurements such as these can be used to increase client confidence and sense of achievement.
- Introduce to peer exercise groups for peer support and encouragement.
- Encourage clients to be more active, e.g. taking stairs instead of lifts.
- Ensure clients also rest adequately in order not to 'burn out'.
- Referral to the GP (for community clients) for primary care management, e.g. prescription for exercise.

Psychological support

- Setting realistic and measurable goals that increase confidence and self-esteem.
- Keeping a food diary to adhere to set diet.
- Change attitudes towards food or drink preparation, e.g. to limit sugar intake.
- Develop problem-solving skills so that clients can have the resources required to sustain a healthy lifestyle.
- Develop links and contacts with self-help and peer support networks.
- Include family/carer who can also offer support and encouragement when at home.
- Weight fluctuates so if weight gain occurs explain this as natural and not a sign of failure. This should be expressed as another challenge, recognizing the client's reality.

Pharmacological treatment

Pharmacological treatment should be evidence based. NICE (2006c) guidance recommends, e.g. Orlistat should be prescribed only as part of an overall plan for managing obesity in adults who meet one of the following criteria:

- BMI of 28.0 kg/m^2 or more with associated risk factors
- BMI of 30.0 kg/m^2 or more

Statin therapy is the gold standard in reducing cholesterol levels as it reduces the amount of cholesterol produced by the liver and stimulates the removal of LDL from circulation (Evered 2007). Statins should also be considered to lower cholesterol. These interventions should also be considered for inpatients who should not be forced to wait for discharge to get this from the GP.

In extreme cases

Bariatric surgery should be considered in line with NICE guidance if everything else has failed to combat weight gain.

Evaluation

Regular review will include

- Measurable targets, used in a before and after comparison:
  - BMI, waist circumference or waist-hip ratio
  - blood pressure
  - blood cholesterol levels
  - client subjective feelings of wellness, mood, self-esteem
- Regular physical checks to screen associated for complications, e.g. BMI or blood tests for diabetes.
- Review of antipsychotic medication if this is directly implicated in weight gain.
- Regular review of the care plan taking into account collateral information from client and carers.

If the client's care changes the review should be completed then, for example, if medication changes, if other complications occur, or if existing complications worsen. The role of community practitioners will include liaison and support with primary care. To monitor physical health NICE (2009) recommends joint care plans and the organization and development of practice case registers for clients with schizophrenia. Community practitioners can help in developing and auditing the effectiveness of such registers.

Physical activity

Box 7.4 Exercise	What are the barriers to physical activity for your clients?

Physical activity has the capacity not only to add years to life, but to bring life to years – through reduced risk of mental disorders, improved quality of life and psychological well-being (DH 2004a). Along with diet and nutrition, it is an important aspect of a healthy lifestyle. However, the prevalence of physical inactivity is high in the UK general population and our client group. This constitutes a challenge to practitioners who may have to motivate, support and encourage clients to exercise who have severe negative symptoms.

Regular physical activity can

- reduce the risk of CHD by up to half;
- reduce the risk of developing type 2 diabetes by 33–50 per cent;
- reduce the risk of dying from cancer;
- reduce the risk of depression and has positive benefits for mental health including reduced anxiety, enhanced mood and self-esteem.

(DH 2002a)

In the UK, NICE guidance on depression (2007b) states that all patients with mild depression should be advised of the benefits of following a structured and supervised exercise programme. Exercise, therefore, is an important factor in mental well-being. The recommended target for physical activity in the UK for adults is at least 30 minutes of at least moderate intensity physical activity a day, on 5 or more days a week (DH 2004a), see Table 7.2.

NICE (2006c) has some basic guidelines when incorporating physical activity into a healthy living plan. They include the following:

- Make enjoyable activities – such as walking, cycling, swimming, aerobics and gardening – part of everyday life.
- Minimize sedentary activities, such as sitting for long periods watching television, at a computer or playing video games.
- Build activity into the working day – for example, use stairs instead of the lift, take a walk at lunchtime.

It is important that physical activity is tailored to client specific needs and capabilities. We must ensure that any exercise plan involves the client and is targeted to meet their wishes and needs. This will involve ensuring their physical safety as well as physical health. This may involve input from a physiotherapist or qualified sports therapist in order that exercise plans take into account individual client needs, for example, safe exercise for clients with movement disorders.

Assessing capability for physical activity

Clients should undergo an assessment before commencing an exercise programme. This is a routine requirement of all gyms. If exercise machines or other sports equipment is used, they should have a thorough induction to prevent accidental injury. A pre-exercise assessment will highlight factors that need to be considered when tailoring an exercise programme and may include those in Table 7.3.

Goals for physical activity must be realistic, achievable and measurable, e.g. 15 minutes of light exercise is realistic, achievable and measurable. Setting achievable goals will increase self confidence. If goals are unrealistic then not achieving them may be demotivating. A good way of socializing for clients would be to go on group walks. Although initially daunting, the increased socializing can increase self confidence and stamina with the added benefit of informal support from others.

While exercise has been shown to improve lipid profiles, glucose tolerance, obesity and hypertension (Connolly and Kelly 2005), Callaghan (2005) states that exercise appears to be a neglected intervention in mental health care. He further notes little or no mention of exercise as a treatment option in most standard mental health/illness texts or reports published by authoritative groups in mental health. Promoting exercise as a non-pharmacological intervention for both physical and mental health problems will be a big challenge for practitioners.

Table 7.2 Recommended physical activity levels

Level	Description	Typical activity pattern	Health benefits
1	Inactive	Always drives to work or takes public transport. Predominantly sedentary job. Minimal household and garden activities. No active recreation.	Nil
2	Lightly active	Will do one or more of: – Some active commuting on foot or by bicycle. – Some walking, lifting and carrying as part of work. – Some undemanding household and gardening activities. – Some active recreation of light intensity.	Some protection against chronic disease. Can be considered a 'stepping stone' to the recommended level (level 3).
3 Recommended level	Moderately active	Will do one or more of: – Regular active commuting on foot or by bicycle. – Regular work-related active tasks – for example, delivering post, household decorator. – Regular household and garden activities. – Regular active recreation or social sport at moderate intensity.	High level of protection against chronic disease. Minimum risk of injury or other adverse health effects.
4	Very active	Will do most of: – Regular active commuting on foot or by bicycle. – Very active job – for example, labourer, farm worker, landscape gardener. – Regular household and garden activities. – Regular active recreation or sport at vigorous intensity.	Maximal protecton against chronic disease. Slight increase in risk of injury and possible some other adverse health effects.
5	Highly active	Performs high volumes of vigorous or very vigorous fitness training, often in order to play vigorous sports.	Maximal protecton against chronic disease. Increased risk of injury and possibly some other adverse health effects.

Source: DH 2004a

Accessing opportunities for physical exercise

While one does not have to join a gym to exercise, doing so can increase the chances of developing social networks. Exercise on referral programmes are used in the UK to promote physical activity. The most common model of exercise referral system is where the GP or practice nurse refers patients to local leisure centres for supervised exercise programmes (DH 2001). Practitioners should act as advocates for clients to ensure that they also have the opportunity to avail of such programmes.

Table 7.3 Example tool for assessing capability for physical activity

Factors	Potential risk
Age	
Cardiovascular	
Respiratory	
Current diabetes status	
Other physical conditions	
Current medication	
Smoking status	
Musculoskeletal function	
Current alcohol intake	
Current exercise levels	
Physical disability	

Box 7.5 **Exercise**	What are the challenges to implementing a healthy eating programme for your client group? How might you overcome these?

Diet and nutrition

It is suggested that positive action on diet and nutrition will contribute to a reduction in preventable deaths from cancer, CHD and stroke (DH 2002a). The UK government has embarked on health education and promotion initiatives designed to educate the general public about healthy eating. Examples of these are 'five a day' – eating at least five portions of fruit and vegetables a day could reduce the risk of deaths from heart disease, stroke and cancer by up to 20 per cent; and advocating a salt intake of no more than 6g per day (DH 2008b).

Relevance to mental health

Our clients have poor diets characterized by a diet high in fat and low in fibre (McCreadie *et al.* 1998; Brown *et al.* 1999). McCreadie (2003) also found that in a sample of clients with SMI, they only consumed 16 portions of fruit and vegetables per week; the DH 2003 recommendation is five a day. Social factors such as finance, lack of motivation or poor knowledge of healthy eating choices may explain this, as it is also a general population problem.

Aims of a healthy diet

Clients and staff should be aware that the aims of a healthy diet are more than just aesthetic. Choice of food and changing eating habits are important. However, the client should be reassured that they can still enjoy a range of foods albeit their preparation may also have to change, e.g. using low salt and sugar alternatives.

Examples of measurable goals include:

- to achieve and maintain glucose control (a normal blood glucose range);
- to achieve and maintain a healthy BMI (BMI 18.5–24.9);

- to achieve and maintain a normal cholesterol level lower than 5mmol/litre for total cholesterol and 3mmol/litre for LDL cholesterol (DH 2000a);
- to have a normal blood pressure and pulse range. British Heart Foundation (2005a) suggest a target blood pressure below 140/85mmHg or if the client has diabetes a target below 130/80mmHg.

General dietary advice

Clients should be encouraged to eat regular meals. Carbohydrates should be a part of each meal as these release energy slowly and keep blood glucose levels stable. This reduces feelings of hunger and the need to snack. High sugar intake should be avoided, e.g. high calorie drinks and snacks should be replaced with sugar free alternatives and fruit. One teaspoon contains five grams of sugar (Peet and Stokes 2004) so intake in tea/coffee should be limited. Sugary snacks such as biscuits, sweets and chocolate should be reduced. This may entail a behaviour change in that clients may eat two or three biscuits with a cup of tea or coffee (containing two or three sugars). If they have five cups of coffee or tea a day then this adds up to one packet of biscuits – on top of their other meals.

Food preparation should include sunflower oil for frying. Foods should be grilled or steamed to reduce cooking with fats. Reducing fried food and take-away food is important especially if clients have diagnosed cardiovascular problems or diabetes. Crisps and nuts may be high in both salt and fat content and should be avoided. Dairy products may need to be fat-free or reduced fat, e.g. skimmed or semi-skimmed milk.

Reducing salt is an effective way of reducing the risk of hypertension. If salt is used in cooking then it should not be used again at the table (double dosing). Processed foods and ready meals should be discouraged as they may have a high salt content: 6g of salt equates to approximately 1 teaspoon.

Clients should be encouraged to eat more vegetables and fruit, aiming for a mixture of at least five portions a day. Food labels can indicate the portion value, but one portion is usually one apple, pear or banana. Fruit juices can also count. However, labels should be checked, as although it might indicate a portion it may also be high in sugar or salt.

NICE (2006c) also recommend strategies such as:

- Eat plenty of fibre-rich foods, such as oats, beans, peas, lentils, grains, seeds, fruit and vegetables, as well as wholegrain bread, and brown rice and pasta.
- Eat a low fat diet and avoid increasing your fat and/or calorie intake.
- Eat breakfast.
- Watch the portion size of meals and snacks, and how often you are eating.
- For adults, minimize the calories you take in from alcohol.

Effects of adverse drug reactions on diet and nutrition

Adverse drug reactions can have consequences for diet and nutrition. These can be very subtle and they may not be as obvious as weight gain, but they are important to consider. Complicating effects of antipsychotics on nutrition outlined by Muir-Cochrane (2006) include

- Anticholinergic potency leading to dry mouth, increased thirst and increased fluid intake
- Hormone system effects leading to fluid retention, thyroid, renal and liver function problems
- Effects on swallowing that compromise nutrition include confusion, delirium, cough, oesophageal ulceration, changes in olfaction and taste, sedation and inattention.

Cultural and religious factors

There are important social determinants in health that go beyond the stereotyped views of the Irish and potatoes or Italians and pasta. Culture and tradition can be powerful influences on nutrition, including food choices and food preparation. Values and beliefs can have an impact on nutritional state, for example, a vegan or vegetarian diet may increase body alkaline content which can be seen during urinalysis testing.

During religious festivals observances such as fasting are required. There are certain days of fasting and abstinence in the Catholic faith where apart from water and medication only one full meal, not containing meat, may be consumed in a twenty-four hour period. In the Muslim faith Ramadan is a holy month where there is a requirement for fasting from dawn to sunset. While people with physical illness can be pardoned from these observances, they may want to participate in them as a matter of faith.

Such fasting will be an important consideration for our clients, especially those with diabetes. The role of the practitioner here is to support and advocate for the client. Practitioners need to involve the dietician and doctor who can advise on foodstuffs to maintain adequate blood glucose levels and modifications to insulin therapy. The inter-professional team will need to discuss the implications for clients with diabetes who want to fast and this should involve input from the client's Imam or appropriate spiritual leader.

Assessing nutritional state

Nutritional assessment aims to increase the client's awareness of a balanced diet, including fluid balance, and to educate them towards healthy eating. It will also highlight deficiencies for which dietary supplements are required. There may be a misleading perception that nutritional assessment is more pertinent in areas such as eating disorders of care of older people. Nutritional assessment is an important aspect of a healthy living programme that should be afforded to all clients, especially those who are at risk of becoming either malnourished or overweight and obese.

Malnourishment

Lean and Wiseman (2008) found that the number of malnourished people leaving NHS hospitals in England had reached almost 140,000 in 2006-7 yet despite this prevalence malnutrition was undiagnosed in up to 70 per cent of patients. They suggest that screening tools are not used routinely and this lack of assessment is a contributing factor in the undiagnosed aspect of this. Holmes (2004) suggests that complications associated with malnourishment cost the NHS around £70 million per year.

Malnourishment is an important part of nutritional screening. It is important that dieticians, especially those experienced in mental health, are involved as they will already be aware of the specific key issues. The Malnutrition Universal Screening Tool (MUST) is commonly used in practice to assess malnutrition. Developed by the British Association of Parenteral and Enteral Nutrition (BAPEN 2003), a risk score is calculated using the client's BMI, unintentional weight loss and illness score. This leads to a low, medium or high risk malnutrition score and advice is given on interventions and treatment.

Skills for assessing nutritional state

Core skills include

- observation
- inspection
- palpation

An underweight or obese person may be identifiable by their appearance. However, BMI or other measurements should be calculated to confirm your observations. Inspection will be required when assessing oral health and palpation when assessing oedema. Client privacy and dignity should always be respected (see Table 7.4).

Social assessment

Poverty is a significant cause of poor dietary choices. Clients may choose to eat to feel full rather than being able to afford to eat well. Due to the effects of their illness, e.g. poor concentration, social isolation or lack of motivation, clients may not have the appropriate social skills needed to cook for themselves. Therefore they may choose convenience food that is usually high in fat, salt and calorie content and low on fruit and vegetables.

Clients may not be able to afford to make healthy food choices as they may not be getting the appropriate benefits. This not only affects food choice but food preparation as they may not have adequate facilities or utensils to cook their own food. A benefits assessment would be valuable in increasing material wealth so that the practitioner can then educate and promote healthy food choices. NICE (2006c) suggest that barriers to lifestyle change include:

- lack of knowledge about buying and cooking food, and how diet and exercise affect health;
- the cost and availability of healthy foods and opportunities for exercise;
- the views of family and community members;
- low levels of fitness, or disabilities;
- low self-esteem and lack of assertiveness.

Fluid balance

Fluid balance is an important homeostatic activity. Fluids are either extracellular (outside cells) or intracellular (inside cells). Fluid balance is maintained through adequate intake and output. The kidneys are the main organs regulating fluid balance and they must produce a minimum of 500–600mL of urine in 24 hours, although normal urinary output is much higher than this (Smith *et al.* 2008a). In the UK a recommendation for fluid intake is an aim to drink at least 1.2 litres of fluid a day (between six to eight glasses) (NHS Direct Wales no date).

Factors that may cause dehydration include

- fever
- diarrhoea
- other gastro-intestinal conditions
- vomiting
- polyuria (in diabetes)
- abuse of laxatives
- taking/abusing diuretics
- adverse drug reaction

Fluid imbalance may occur due to decreased intake, or increased output. Electrolyte imbalance,

Table 7.4 Assessment of nutritional state

Assessment	Criteria	Possible physical cause
Physical appearance	Under-weight, overweight, obese – check BMI **(I)**	Anaemia
	General weakness and lethargy **(O)**	Diabetes
	Ill-fitting clothes may be a sign of recent weight gain **(O)**	Malnutrition
	Baggy clothes may be used to camouflage weight loss **(O)**	Fluid and electrolyte imbalance
	Waist measurement **(I)**	
	Waist–hip ratio measurement **(I)**	Heart failure, cancer, starvation
	Abdominal ascites – fluid in the peritoneal cavity (McFerran 2008) **(O) (I) (P)**	
Skin	Skin may be flaky or dry **(O) (I)**	Vitamin deficiency
	Hair and nails may be brittle **(O) (I)**	
	Slow healing wounds **(O) (I)**	
Cardiovascular	May be signs of oedema in the ankles or wrists **(O) (I) (P)**	Heart block, fluid imbalance
	Goitre **(O) (I) (P)**	Iodine deficiency
Respiratory	Breathlessness associated with excess weight **(O)**	Obesity, orthopnoea
Oral health	Mouth ulcers, sores on the tongue or bleeding gums **(O) (I)**	Vitamin C deficiency
	Pear drop smell on breath **(O)**	Diabetes
Blood tests	Low full blood count results will indicate conditions such as, increased cholesterol levels, abnormal glucose levels or poor thyroid function **(I)**	Anaemia, vitamin B deficiency Poor diet, sedentary lifestyle Endocrine disorder
Urinalysis	Ketones may indicate severe dieting, low pH – starvation, glucose – diabetes **(I)**	Renal problems, special diet, diabetes
Neurological	Presence of tremor or nystagmus **(O) (P)**	Vitamin B deficiency
	Night blindness **(I)**	Vitamin A deficiency
	Confusion or delirium **(O)**	Dehydration, electrolyte imbalance
Psychological	Low self-esteem due to body image, poor concentration, demotivation **(O) (I)**	Possible depression, anaemia, vitamin deficiency
Mobility	May be reduced due to excess weight, or a lack of energy stemming from poor diet, oedema may be present which affects mobility, if underweight may be too weak to move **(O)**	Low calcium levels, Insufficient protein in diet
Family history of obesity	There may be genetic predisposition to obesity (Loos and Bouchard 2003), past medical history of diabetes	

(O) = Observation, **(I)** = Inspection, **(P)** = Palpation

where toxins that need to be expelled are retained in the body, is a complication. Electrolyte imbalance can lead to delirium and confusion, which in some client groups may be mistaken for symptoms of the mental illness, e.g. dementia. However, this can be a life-threatening event and in vulnerable clients should be closely monitored. Urinalysis will help indicate potential fluid balance problems.

Dehydration and electrolyte imbalance can affect cardiac and renal system functions (Scales and Pilsworth 2008). Symptoms of dehydration include

- thirst
- dry mouth
- dried or chapped lips
- dry, flaky skin
- reduced urine output
- concentrated urine
- tachycardia
- confusion

Dehydrated clients should be placed on a fluid balance chart to monitor input and output. All ingested fluids, either orally or by IV infusion are recorded against outputs. Outputs should be safely collected using a bedpan, urinal bottle or catheter and measured. If a urinalysis test is done it should be remembered that stale urine may give a false-positive reading for high pH or bilirubinuria. Remember the client's dignity and respect during the process of collecting outputs. If a client is catheterized then the catheter bag will have a measurement scale that can be easily observed. It is very important that measurements are accurately recorded and documented.

Diuretics may be prescribed for clients with cardiovascular problems so that excess fluids can be expelled from the body. This should be considered if a client complains of frequency of micturation. If they do not take diuretics and complain of frequency of micturation, then this might be a sign of diabetes mellitus.

Overhydration can also be a problem for the body and this may occur due to

- polydipsia (in diabetes)
- heart failure
- renal impairment
- liver disease

(Scales and Pilsworth 2008)

Another cause of overhydration is a phenomenon where clients develop a compulsion to drink water in excess. Singh *et al.* (1985) report a case of a client with delusional beliefs who drank excessive amounts of water as a religious offering. Overhydration can lead to water intoxication, which is different to polydipsia as described earlier, but more akin to dipsomania – a compulsion to drink alcohol to excess (see Ferrier 1985). Overhydration can lead to hyponatraemia, a condition where there are low levels of sodium in the blood due to dilution by excess water intake. However, severe vomiting or diarrhoea can also cause it.

Treating overhydration will depend on the primary cause. If it is secondary to a heart condition then the heart condition should be effectively treated and managed. This may include the prescription of a diuretic to help with elimination of excess fluids. If the cause is related to diabetes mellitus then this will also require treatment.

Box 7.6 Exercise   In relation to your client group, what would you describe as the biggest challenges regarding nutrition and diet?

Diabetes

Homeostasis of glucose control

Diabetes occurs due to an imbalance in the levels of glucose and insulin in the blood. The Islets of Langerhans in the pancreas has alpha and beta cells. The alpha cells secrete 'glucagon' which functions to increase the blood level of glucose and the beta cells secrete 'insulin' which functions to decrease blood levels of glucose and increase utilization of glucose. Blood glucose levels control secretion of glucagon and insulin.

Having a balanced diet is important for maintaining effective diabetes control as it will help to maintain blood-glucose within a set target range and reduce the risk of complications such as hypoglycaemic coma. Good nutrition will also reduce the risk of complications of diabetes.

What we know about diabetes

It seems that diabetes, especially type 2 diabetes (T2D), has become an epidemic in western society. T2D is a major public health concern, especially in people at younger ages. In 2000 the World Health Organization estimated the worldwide prevalence of diabetes at 171,000,000 with an estimated prevalence of 366,000,000 by 2030 (WHO 2000a).

In a national context the prevalence of diabetes in the UK is 3.6 per cent, around 2.3 million people (Diabetes UK 2007) with an estimated prevalence of more than 2.5 million by 2010 (DH 2006). However, T2D is largely a 'silent' illness and there may be up to 1,000,000 people unaware that they have it. Holt (2005) suggests that the onset of diabetes predates actual diagnosis by around a decade.

Diabetes has great impacts on society. In terms of health care costs, diabetes accounted for 5 per cent of all NHS expenditure in 2002, with an estimated annual cost of £1.3 billion pounds (DH 2006b). However, there are greater impacts on individual suffers and their families/ carers. Life expectancy for sufferers is reduced by 5–7 years for T2D; there is a greater risk of stroke and heart problems; and around 30 per cent of patients with T2D develop kidney disease (DH 2006b).

What we know about diabetes in people with mental illness

While it is recognized that our clients have a greater risk of developing diabetes than the general population, the process of this is very complex. Research shows the following:

- The prevalence of diabetes in people with schizophrenia is generally estimated at between 2–4 per cent (Bushe and Holt 2004).
- People with schizophrenia are a high risk group for abnormal glucose homeostasis (Gough 2005).
- Clients with bipolar disorder appear to be at greater risk of developing T2D. A US study by Cassidy *et al.* (1999) estimated the prevalence at almost 3 times that for the general population.

A survey by the Disability Rights Commission (DRC 2006) found that 41 per cent of those with schizophrenia and diabetes are diagnosed under the age of 55, compared with 30 per cent of others with diabetes; and 19 per cent of people with diabetes who have schizophrenia have died, as have 4 per cent of people with bipolar disorder, compared with 9 per cent of people with no serious mental health problems. These statistics show that our clients not only develop diabetes at younger ages than the general population, but also that their prognosis is often poorer.

Diabetes is under-diagnosed in our clients and the first time it is encountered may be in respect of a clinical incident, e.g. diabetic ketoacidosis or a hypoglycaemic coma. This may be because signs and symptoms are conflated with adverse drug reactions, for example, increased fluid intake may be mistaken as a response for dry mouth but not seen as polydipsia in diabetes.

Causes of diabetes in our clients

The causes of T2D in our clients are very complex. The risk of getting T2D in our client group, especially schizophrenia, is higher than the general population (Dixon *et al.* 2000). The causes of T2D are similar to that of the general population – sedentary lifestyles, poor diet and lack of exercise which contribute to obesity and impaired glucose tolerance. The complexity arises when we include adverse drug reactions, especially new atypical drugs such as clozapine and olanzapine, which are most commonly associated with increased rates of obesity and diabetes (Healy 2005). However, Kohen (2004) notes that in the late 1950s there were reports that chlorpromazine was linked to hyperglycaemia, glycosuria and weight gain.

Does atypical medication cause T2D? A review by Smith *et al.* (2008b) found newer atypical medications have a 30 per cent increased risk of diabetes compared with typical medications. However, they suggest that this result is treated with caution. Smith *et al.*'s review shows that any evidence for such a link is poor but suggest that clinicians 'implement protocols for identifying physical illnesses, in particular diabetes, in people with schizophrenic illnesses' (p. 410). However, Healy (2005) suggests that olanzapine and clozapine raise blood lipid levels and blood glucose levels, which leads to diabetes.

Insulin resistance is another metabolic disorder defined as a disease process whereby an individual becomes resistant to their inherent insulin production (Jeffery (2003). Risk factors for insulin resistance include

- obesity
- high waist-hip ratio (apple shaped rather than pear shaped)
- hypertension
- family history of T2D or cardiovascular disease
- ethnicity
- gestational diabetes
- smoking

(Jeffery 2003)

Screening for and identifying T2D

Practitioners should be aware of the risk factors for T2D (see Table 7.5). Standard 2 of the *National Service Framework for Diabetes* (DH 2001b) aims to identify people who do not yet know

Table 7.5 Modifiable and non-modifiable risk factors and associated disorders for type 2 diabetes

Modifiable risk factors	Non-modifiable risk factors
Overweight and obesity (as measured by BMI)	Ethnicity
Sedentary lifestyle	Family history of T2D
Previously identified glucose intolerance – impaired glucose tolerance or impaired fasting glucose	Age
Metabolic syndrome: • Hypertension • Decreased HDL cholesterol • Increased triglycerides	Gender History of gestational diabetes Polycystic ovary syndrome
Dietary factors	
Intrauterine environment	
Inflammation	

Source: Alberti *et al.* (2007)

that they have diabetes. Health education and promotion can then be employed to reduce the complications of diabetes from arising. Practitioners should be observant for the common symptoms of T2D, for example, excessive thirst, frequent micturition, lethargy or unplanned weight loss. If these are present then a blood sample should be taken and sent for screening.

Diagnosing diabetes

When testing a blood sample, the normal fasting blood glucose level is 3.3–6.1 mmol/l. Diabetes UK (2008b) gives the following levels as indicators of diabetes:

- a random venous plasma glucose concentration ≥11.1 mmol/l; or
- a fasting plasma glucose concentration ≥7.0 mmol/l (whole blood ≥6.1mmol/l); or
- two hour plasma glucose concentration ≥11.1 mmol/l two hours after an oral glucose tolerance test.

The risk factors for T2D are outlined in Table 7.6.

If we put this in the context of our clients we can prioritize screening to the following:

- those with current heart disease or who have suffered a stroke;
- those over 40 years old;
- those with a family history of diabetes;
- those with a BMI of 30+; or
- those with a waist size greater than 88cm (female) or 102cm (male); and
- overweight children or young people in Child and Adolescent Mental Health Services.

Managing T2D

Changing lifestyle factors is a key strategy, by

Table 7.6 Screening for T2D

Screening variable	Risk factor
Medical history	CHD, CVD, stroke
Blood pressure	If you have diabetes, kidney disease or heart disease a target BP is below 130/80mmHg (BHF 2005)
Presence of noticeable symptoms	Polydipsia, polyuria
Urinalysis	Specific gravity, glycosuria
Overweight or obese	BMI greater than 25.9 or waist measurement >94cm (>37 inches) for white and black men, and >90cm (>35 inches) for Asian men, and >80cm (>31.5 inches) for white, black and Asian women (Diabetes UK 2008)
Sedentary lifestyle	Low exercise or physical activity
Social	Family member with diabetes
Metabolic Syndrome Markers	High HDL cholesterol Hypertension
Demographic factors – age and culture	White and >40 or ethnic minority – African-Caribbean, Asian
Diagnosis of schizophrenia	Linked to increased risk of diabetes
Taking 'high risk' medications	Olanzapine, clozapine

- increasing physical activity
- regulating diet
- stopping smoking
- reducing alcohol intake
- regular monitoring of blood glucose levels

Pharmacological treatment

Alberti *et al.* (2007) suggest that pharmacological interventions for the prevention of diabetes are recommended as a secondary intervention either to follow lifestyle interventions or in conjunction with them. If lifestyle factors are not enough to regain glycaemic control then medication may be prescribed to achieve this. The most common medication is a hypoglycaemic agent such as metformin, which is widely accepted as the first line drug (Heine *et al.* 2006). However, this drug may be contraindicated in clients with renal damage so should be considered with caution in clients taking lithium. Medication should not be used as a substitute for changing lifestyle factors.

Checklist prior to commencing an atypical antipsychotic

The medications with the high risk of weight gain are olanzapine and clozapine. Quetiapine, and risperidone pose a moderate risk while amisulpride a low risk (Taylor *et al.* 2005). Clients should be screened prior to commencing or changing antipsychotic medication. There is no hard and fast timescale but Table 7.7 below illustrates one. This allows for accurate assessment of weight gain and screening for potential health risks, e.g. cardiac problems or diabetes.

Complications of T2D

Delayed diagnosis leads to a prolonged exposure to untreated symptoms increasing the risk of complications. T2D is notable for the increased cardiovascular risk that it carries for coronary artery disease (leading to heart attacks, angina), peripheral artery disease (leg claudication, gangrene) and carotid artery disease (strokes, dementia) (NICE 2008). Diabetes is one of the major causes of blindness, kidney failure and amputation (Marks 2003).

Watkins (2003) outlines the factors increasing the risk of developing CHD in diabetic patients as smoking, hypertension, insulin resistance, Asian origin, microalbuminuria, diabetic

Table 7.7 Metabolic screening for antipsychotic medication

	On commencing or changing medication	Week 8	Week 16	6 Monthly	Yearly (or as required)
Clinical variable					
Blood pressure					
Pulse					
Body mass index					
Waist measurement					
Blood tests – FBC, fasting glucose, cholesterol levels, liver function					
Urinalysis					
ECG					

nephropathy, poor glycaemic control and hyperlipidaemia. In respect of our client group this gives us an indication of who we can effectively target with appropriate interventions and treatment.

Health education and health promotion

We will have a key role in prevention of T2D through health education and promotion in the areas of nutrition, diet and physical activity. The process will be inter-professional and will involve team members such as dietician, occupational therapist (OT), exercise therapist and carer/family. The OT and dietician could arrange educational shopping trips to supermarkets where they can educate clients about healthy eating while they do their shopping. Food labelling can be very confusing so the dietician would help in explaining food labels to clients, highlighting the healthy alternatives and cautioning on foods that have a high salt and sugar content.

Primary prevention

Primary prevention aims to prevent the condition arising in the first place. Following on from screening, the aim for clients who do not test positive for a metabolic disorder is to prevent them from getting one. This will include practical aspects of health education and promotion, advice on healthy diet, nutrition and physical activity. A review of diabetes risk related to medication regime should also be considered.

Secondary prevention

Secondary prevention aims to identify conditions early so that interventions can be tailored as soon as possible. This will reduce the potential for complications developing and delay the progression of the condition.

As a result of screening, clients may be identified as having T2D. Here the practitioner would be following the process as laid out in primary prevention, but the client may need some adjunct treatment to help with the process, e.g. a referral to a diabetes nurse specialist or prescription of an oral hypoglycaemic agent. Clients that smoke should be offered a referral to smoking cessation services.

Tertiary prevention

Tertiary prevention is employed when the condition has already been diagnosed. Here the aim is to improve the quality of life of the client and reduce the impact of the condition in daily life. Tertiary prevention will be required for clients who have developed diabetes and have suffered a physical illness as a result of this, e.g. heart attack or stroke. Here the practitioner's role is to support the client and enable them to adapt their lifestyle. The aim here is to increase the quality of the client's life following a significant disabling event.

Metabolic syndrome

Metabolic syndrome is a cluster of several risk factors for heart disease. While there is no unique definition of metabolic syndrome, the diagnostic criteria defined by the WHO (1999) are the presence of T2D, impaired glucose tolerance, insulin resistance, together with two or more of the following:

- dyslipidaemia – low HDL cholesterol and high triglycerides;
- hypertension – blood pressure >140/90mmHg;

- obesity with high BMI;
- micro-albuminuria.

Additional associated abnormalities may include hyperuricaemia and polycystic ovary syndrome. The following deciphers this definition. Dyslipidaemia is a disorder of lipid (fat) metabolism and is usually hyperlipidaemia – high cholesterol. The normal range of cholesterol in the blood would be lower than 5mmol/litre for total cholesterol and 3mmol/litre for LDL cholesterol (DH 2000a). High density lipoproteins (HDL) protect against CHD as they decrease risk factors such as atherosclerosis by 'cleaning' excess lipids from the arteries and carrying them to the liver where they are broken down. Increased triglyceride levels are linked to atherosclerosis, which increases the risk of CHD and stroke. Micro-albuminuria (MA) is the presence of of small amounts of albumin in the urine. If urinalysis proves positive for glucose a sample should be sent for analysis to determine if MA is present. MA has been associated with an elevated risk of serious cardiovascular events including stroke (Ovbiagele 2008). Hyperuricaemia is increased levels of uric acid in the blood. Polycystic ovary syndrome affects women and symptoms include enlarged ovaries with small cysts (McFerran 2008). This is associated with insulin resistance and obesity.

Risk factors for metabolic syndrome

Tonkin *et al.* (2003) suggest a prevalence of up to 25 per cent in the UK population. Holt (2005) suggests that central obesity – fat deposited around the abdomen – places the individual at a greater risk of developing it. The prevalence of metabolic syndrome is higher in certain groups:

- ethnic subgroups, e.g. Asian and African Caribbean
- women with polycystic ovary disease
- patients with schizophrenia
- people with non-alcoholic fatty liver disease

Clinical implications of having metabolic syndrome include a threefold increase in risk for coronary heart disease and stroke compared to individuals with normal glucose tolerance (British Nutrition Foundation 2004).

Treatment of metabolic syndrome

Treatment should begin with primary prevention. At risk clients should be screened and if they are clear they should be given health education and promotion advice around healthy lifestyles and exercise. However, Barnes *et al.* (2007) found rates of screening of metabolic syndrome to be well below recommended levels in an audit of Assertive Outreach Teams.

For clients with metabolic syndrome the emphasis should be on secondary prevention, e.g. preventing complications and effective management. Treatment of main risk factors should be prioritized and will include pharmacological and non-pharmacological interventions. These should be explained as treatment interventions not lifestyle choices.

- Pharmacotherapy, e.g. statins (cholesterol-lowering drugs) may be indicated for dyslipidaemia, elevated triglycerides and low HDL may also need medication.
- Lifestyle changes may be made, e.g. a weight management plan to reduce excess body fat, reducing calorie intake, saturated fats and sodium.
- The client should be encouraged to increase fruit and vegetables in the diet and to exercise, especially exercise that involves increased heart and lung activity.

What can the MHN do to promote healthy eating and exercise?

Health education and health promotion are good starting points. Practitioners should give as much information on positive health as possible and at every opportunity. This should be in a constructive and empowering way as clients may feel powerless or unable to change. In this sense it is important that education is not just about eating healthily, but also about cognitive-behavioural strategies designed to inhibit negative perceptions clients have about themselves.

Changing behaviours will entail changing attitudes – in practitioners as much as clients. We should dispense with the 'you can't teach an old dog new tricks' idea. Negative staff attitudes can be as much a barrier to change as client demotivation. We should be increasing clients' awareness of healthy eating and exercise, opportunities to engage in lifestyle changes and peer support groups in the community. Information should be presented in a way that is accessible for clients and carers.

Box 7.7	Look at the vending machines located inside or near your ward. How healthy are the
Exercise	food and drink choices available to clients?

Providing choice is a mantra in health policy. In inpatient areas clients should be given the choice of fruit and vegetables as often as possible. A simple audit of vending machines in mental health units will indicate that healthy food choices for clients are limited. There will most likely be the conciliatory piece of fruit there but the quantity of fruit will not be the same in proportion to chocolate bars, crisps or sweets. Drink machines will most often have high calorie drinks also.

Exercise is a non-pharmacological way of managing both physical and mental health problems. Practitioners should encourage clients to participate in exercise programmes – both in hospital and the community. We will need to be creative in how we present these as interventions as well as lifestyle choices. If we are too evangelical then clients may not feel supported to engage. We should enable clients to express their own ideas for exercise and lifestyle choices and empower them to follow these as goals. Mostly we should be there to support them and to monitor the effects of lifestyle on physical health.

Conclusions

Making moderate changes in lifestyles can result in considerable gains. For example, by reducing saturated fat intake and increasing exercise we can reduce the risk of heart disease. Regular physical activity reduces the risk of breast and colon cancer and possibly that of endometrial and prostate cancer (WHO 2003).

The WHO (2003) also suggests advice on ways of changing daily nutritional intake and increasing energy expenditure by:

- reducing energy-rich foods high in saturated fat and sugar;
- cutting the amount of salt in the diet;
- increasing the amount of fresh fruit and vegetables in the diet;
- undertaking moderate-intensity physical activity for at least an hour a day.

The dietary changes that clients require should not be drastic; they should be planned, SMART (Specific, Measurable, Attainable, Realistic and Timely) changes. The main factor is adopting a 'healthy' diet but this may be difficult for clients living in socially deprived areas. Therefore part of the overall assessment should be a social assessment to ensure that the client and carers have the appropriate benefits level to support lifestyle change.

A shift in attitudes is the biggest challenge. But this sword cuts both ways. Changing attitudes of clients towards healthy lifestyles incorporating smoking cessation, dietary changes and exercise is as important as changing staff attitudes that stigmatize clients as being unable to change, or that physical health is not their remit.

Summary of key points

- Practitioners should engage clients in adopting a healthy lifestyle by using government public health initiatives as means of modifying diet and physical activity.
- Clients should be routinely screened for metabolic conditions such as T2D.
- Assessment of diet, nutrition and physical activity should include socio-economic factors that might inhibit lifestyle change as well as physical and psychological factors.
- Weight management and physical activity programmes should be offered to all clients, but especially those on atypical antipsychotics that cause weight gain.
- Practitioners should involve clients and carers in plans to develop healthy lifestyles and physical activity regimes.

Quick quiz

1 What is the UK government recommendation for physical activity for adults?
2 How do you calculate (a) body mass index and (b) waist-hip ratio?
3 What are the WHO diagnostic criteria for (a) underweight, (b) overweight and (c) obesity?
4 What are high density lipoproteins and what function do they serve?
5 What is glycosuria and how might it be detected?

8 Medication, adverse drug reactions and physical health

By the end of this chapter you will be able to:

- Describe common neurotransmitters and their effects
- Describe some of the physical adverse drug reactions of psychotropic medications on – metabolism, the cardiac system, sexual dysfunction and severe drug reactions
- Examine issues of non-compliance stemming from physical adverse drug reactions
- Examine the assessment and monitoring of physical adverse drug reactions
- Explore the role of practitioners in limiting the disabilities caused by adverse drug reactions

Introduction

**Box 8.1
Exercise**   What are the common adverse drug reactions (ADRs) of typical and atypical antipsychotics?

Since the 1950s medication has been a mainstay in the treatment of mental illness. The development of chlorpromazine is often credited with the advent of community care as more people with mental illness could be treated at home instead of hospital. However, what was apparent then, as now, is that psychotropic drugs have serious side effects. In some cases these constitute a high risk to clients' physical health. For example, in 1949 Cade, an Australian psychiatrist, found that lithium was effective in treating mania, however, in 1949 lithium was banned by the US Food and Drug Administration due to deaths in patients with cardiac disease (Keltner and Folks 2005).

This chapter will include the blood as an integral part of the cardiac system as some adverse drug reactions are blood dyscrasias – abnormalities in blood cell production – which can have serious implications in a client's ability to fight infection.

What does the brain do?

The brain is a complex organ forming an integral part of the central nervous system (CNS). It is responsible for

- maintaining homeostasis
- regulating basic needs, e.g. hunger and sleep
- regulating drives and impulses
- regulating and interpreting emotions
- enabling us to think
- controlling responses to a range of sensory stimuli
- enabling us to process, store and recall data
- enabling us to initiate and respond in communication
- giving us drive and motivation
- storing and recalling memory (may be selective)

It contains nerve cells called neurones of which there are three types:

- sensory – neurones that carry information from the sense organs to the CNS;
- motor – neurones that carry information from the CNS to the muscles and glands; and
- interneurones – which connect neurones to other neurones.

(Gross 2005)

Neurotransmitters

Neurones communicate with each other through a combination of electrical impulses and chemical messengers called neurotransmitters. Chemical neurotransmission is the process involving the release of a neurotransmitter by one neurone and the binding of that neurotransmitter to a receptor on another neurone (Kaplan and Sadock 1994). Table 8.1 gives an outline of the neurotransmitters important in psychiatry. An excess or lack of these can contribute to mental and physical health problems.

Why 'physical' adverse drug reactions?

Surely ADRs are physical? The purpose here is not to examine traditional movement related disorders. With the noticeable rise of ADRs such as obesity, T2D, dyslipidaemia and coronary problems, a less traditional focus is appropriate. ADRs are a unique risk factor for our clients as they contribute to metabolic and cardiovascular conditions and early death.

Psychotropic medications can have adverse effects on our major body systems and activities of daily living:

- Cardiac system – prolonged QT interval and cardiac dysrrhythmias
- Alimentary system – oral health problems affecting chewing and taste, weight gain and constipation
- CNS depression which might affect receptiveness to pain which may be a reason for under-reporting physical illness, e.g. clients may not feel toothache until it is very severe and the tooth and gums are badly infected
- Activities of daily living – loss of appetite, loss of libido, insomnia, mobility

Although some ADRs are 'rare', it is important that we are aware of them so that we can react swiftly and confidently if we encounter them.

Why monitor ADRs?

Waddington *et al.* (1998) found that receiving more than one antipsychotic concurrently was associated with reduced survival in people with schizophrenia. Therefore monitoring ADRs is

Table 8.1 Common neurotransmitters, their functions and effects in mental health

Neurotransmitter	Function	Psychological effect	Physical effect
Dopamine	Stimulates the heart Controls muscle and motor coordination Stimulates the hypothalamus to release hormones	Increased levels may contribute to schizophrenia and mania Decreased levels may contribute to depression, Parkinson's disease	Hyperprolactinaemia, hypertension and tachycardia
Acetylcholine	Plays a role in memory and learning Regulates mood, aggressive and sexual behaviour Stimulates the parasympathetic nervous system	Increased levels may contribute to depression Decreased levels may contribute to Alzheimer's disease, Huntington's chorea, Parkinson's disease	Dry mouth, blurred vision, constipation and tachycardia, confusion, memory and concentration problems
Noradrenaline	Regulates mood, attention and arousal Stimulates the 'fight or flight' response	Increased levels may contribute to mania Decreased levels may contribute to depression	Orthostatic hypotension, tachycardia, dizziness, priapism
Serotonin	Regulates attention, behaviour, sleep, body temperature, hunger, aggression and pain perception	Increased levels may contribute to anxiety Decreased levels may contribute to depression	Weight gain, hypotension, decreased appetite, headaches
Histamine	Inflammatory response, alertness and gastric secretion	–	Some antipsychotics block histamine receptors and this causes increased sedation and weight gain
Gaba-aminobutyric acid (GABA)	Reduces anxiety, excitation and aggression Anticonvulsant and muscle relaxing properties	Increased levels may contribute to reducing anxiety Decreased levels may contribute to mania, anxiety and schizophrenia	Low seizure threshold

Source: Adapted from Varchol and Raynor 2008

an important role for practitioners because it is good practice for clients taking medications. Monitoring ADRs has become more complex as we now need to be aware of a wider range of negative effects. It is also compulsory for medicines such as clozapine and lithium, where we need to ensure client safety. Finally, monitoring ADRs is a way of determining how effective medications are in helping clients to recover.

How do psychotropic medications work?

Little is known about the action of drugs on neurotransmitter activity. What *is* known is that psychotropic drugs act on different receptor sites, including those that they are not designed to work on. A simplistic biological theory is neurotransmitter excess or deficiency. Too much, or not enough, neurotransmitter can lead to mental health problems (see Table 8.1). However, such is the nature of psychotropic medications that they may alleviate symptoms but they also cause numerous ADRs.

The process of neurotransmission is affected by most drugs used in psychiatry (Kaplan and Sadock 1994). Psychotropic medications work by manipulating the action of neurotransmitters. This manipulation can be in the following ways:

- Typical antipsychotics block dopamine and acetylcholine receptors.
- Atypical antipsychotics block dopamine and serotonin receptors.
- Antidepressants block re-uptake of neurotransmitters such as serotonin and inhibit the enzyme monoamine oxadise which destroys neurotransmitters such as serotonin and noradrenaline.
- Mood stabilizers such as lithium interfere with neurotransmitter activity both in synthesis and re-uptake. It may also promote electrical stability.
- Benzodiazepines facilitate the transmission of gamma amino-butyric acid GABA, which helps inhibit (relax) brain activity by slowing responses to stimuli.

ADRs in psychotropic medication

Box 8.2
Exercise   List the typical and atypical antipsychotics used in your clinical area.

Antipsychotic medications

Antipsychotic medications act primarily on positive symptoms of schizophrenia such as delusions and hallucinations. Their effectiveness in treating more problematic negative symptoms is questionable. Antipsychotics are usually divided into two types: traditional antipsychotics, such as haloperidol and chlorpromazine, referred to as **typical antipsychotics**; and the newer antipsychotics, such as olanzapine and clozapine, referred to as **atypical antipsychotics**.

Antipsychotics have a range of ADRs that can appear at any time after commencement of treatment and are usually dose-effect related. This means they become more severe with higher doses. The main difference between typical and atypical antipsychotics is their range of ADRs.

Typical antipsychotics

Typical antipsychotics come in two types of potency:

- Low-potency antipsychotics normally require large doses and can cause sedation.
- High-potency antipsychotics usually require lower doses and tend to cause more movement disorders.

ADRs commonly associated with typical antipsychotics that we usually assess for include the following:

- Tardive dyskinesia: involuntary muscle movements, e.g. tremor (tongue, hands), tongue protrusion, chewing movements
- Acute dystonic reactions: muscle spasm in neck and back, oculogyric crisis

- Akathisia: involuntary motor restlessness
- Parkinsonian symptoms: excess salivation, cogwheel rigidity, shuffling gait
- Anti-cholinergic effects: sedation, dry mouth, blurred vision and constipation

Atypical antipsychotic medications

Atypical antipsychotics are the recognized front line treatment for schizophrenia in the UK (NICE 2002). ADRs associated with atypical antipsychotics include

- metabolic and weight gain
- cardiac system effects
- blood dyscrasias
- sexual dysfunction

These do not represent the only ADRs but they are important risk variables in provoking physical conditions that lead to early death or non-compliance in clients. Most ADRs usually recede with time and without the use of any adjunct medication. Interventions for managing adverse effects include

- Non-pharmacological: lifestyle changes, healthy living programmes, dietary changes and increasing fluid intake for constipation and dry mouth;
- Pharmacological: prescription of adjunct medications to counteract ADRs, altering the dose of medication, stopping or changing medications.

Antipsychotic drugs can produce metabolic disorders that require treatment with 'physical' care medications, e.g. metformin is a drug used in the management of T2D. Williams and Pinfold (2006) in a survey for Rethink, a UK mental health charity, found the most disturbing ADRs reported by clients were:

- sedation and lethargy 22 per cent
- weight gain 19 per cent
- shaking and tremors 6 per cent
- sexual dysfunction 3 per cent

Worryingly, they also found that 54 per cent of the sample did not receive any written information about ADRs. For most clients disabling ADRs are usually associated with traditional drugs, however, new evidence suggests that metabolic abnormalities with atypical medications are a concern for clients.

ADRs are not limited to typical or atypical generations of drugs. For example, tardive dyskinesia has been reported in clozapine (Novartis 2008) and risperidone (Janssen Pharmaceuticals 2008) and blood dyscrasias, i.e. agranulocytosis, can occur with typical antipsychotics like chlorpromazine (BNF 2007).

Antidepressants

There are three main types of antidepressant medication; tricyclics, selective serotonin reuptake inhibitors (SSRIs) and monoamine oxidase inhibitors (MAOIs). All antidepressant drugs increase serotonin function and may also increase noradrenaline function (Gelder *et al.* 1996).

Tricyclic antidepressants

These are referred to as 'older' antidepressants. These can be fatal in overdose due to their cardiotoxic nature (Patton 2008). They tend to have more ADRs than 'newer' antidepressants including

- arrhythmias
- heart block
- orthostatic hypotension
- galactorrhoea
- agranulocytosis
- hyponatraemia
- urinary retention

(BNF 2007)

Selective serotonin reuptake inhibitors

These are referred to as 'newer' antidepressants. They act by blocking the reuptake of serotonin (hence their name). Increased levels of serotonin reduce feelings of depression. ADRs include:

- angio-oedema
- galactorrhoea
- urticaria
- gastrointestinal effects
- hepatitis
- jaundice
- withdrawal effects

(BNF 2007)

It may take weeks before clients notice any positive effects. This slow response may lead clients to think that the medication is not working and to stop taking it. Perceived non-effect is an important factor in non-compliance.

Monoamine oxidase inhibitors (MAOIs)

MAOIs act by blocking the enzymes that destroy neurotransmitters such as noradrenalin and serotonin. Blocking these enzymes enables neurotransmitters to accumulate and remain active for longer, alleviating depressive symptoms.

Clients taking MAOIs are required to make compulsory dietary changes. This is due to the potential interaction between MAOIs and tyramine which can release neurotransmitters such as dopamine and noradrenaline. This interaction can provoke cardiac problems. Foods high in tyramine need to be avoided and include pickled herring, mature cheese, cured meats, drinks based on yeast extracts, overripe fruit and red wine. Bananas may be taken in small quantities but if a severe headache or symptoms of hypertension occur these should be immediately assessed.

Mood stabilizers

Lithium is a mainstay treatment for bipolar affective disorder and mania. However, the action of lithium is poorly understood. Varchol and Raynor (2008) suggest that lithium as a positively charged ion acts by stabilizing electrical activity in neurones. Lithium has a narrow therapeutic range making it easy for clients to suffer adverse effects. If these go undiagnosed lithium toxicity may occur which can have serious implications for clients. Lithium toxicity is related to the concentration of lithium in blood plasma. However, side effects of lithium toxicity can occur even within therapeutic levels. The therapeutic range of lithium is 0.4–1mmol/l (BNF 2007).

Benzodiazepines

Benzodiazepines are referred to as anxiolytics and are used in conjunction with antipsychotics in rapid tranquillization. ADRs include cardiac effects such as low blood pressure, light-headedness and muscle weakness. Another significant problem with benzodiazepines is addiction which can lead to severe withdrawal effects. This is why a gradual withdrawal regime is required. Ability to perform motor tasks, e.g. driving, is also impaired as reaction times are slowed down.

Metabolic ADRs with medication

Psychotropic medications are associated with metabolic reactions that can increase the risk of coronary events. Such is the extent of metabolic reactions that these are referred to as the 'new' tardive dyskinesia. Taylor *et al.* (2005) state that common metabolic reactions include

- hyperlipidaemia
- increased low density lipoproteins (bad cholesterol)
- decreased high density lipoproteins (good cholesterol)
- increased triglycerides
- T2D
- obesity or severe weight gain

Metabolic ADRs are features of most antipsychotic (typical and atypical) medications as they may affect histamine and serotonin receptors and this can cause sedation and weight gain (Taylor *et al.* 2005). The development of diabetes in clients taking olanzapine and Clozaril seems to be an effect of treatment that is independent of weight gain (Healy 2005). However, there is an increasing recognition that severe mental illness may represent an independent risk factor for diabetes (Expert Consensus Group 2005). Routine metabolic monitoring does not occur in our clients, even though they have higher rates of diabetes and an increased exposure to metabolic risk factors. There is a lack of coherent policy framework for metabolic screening and monitoring with confusion around whose role it should be.

Second generation antipsychotics and metabolic abnormalities

Most atypical antipsychotics produce weight gain and some are also implicated in diabetes and dyslipidaemia, for example:

- Olanzapine and clozapine produce weight gain, risk of diabetes and worsening lipid profile.
- Risperidone and quetiapine produce weight gain but there are discrepant results for diabetes and worsening lipid profile.
- Aripiprazole and Ziprasidone produce minimal weight gain and have no effect on diabetes or lipid profile.

(American Diabetes Association, American Psychiatric Association, American Association of Clinical Endocrinologists, North American Association for the Study of Obesity 2004)

Box 8.3 Exercise   List your client's medications and examine the potential cardiac adverse reactions.

Obesity and weight gain

Causes of obesity, diabetes and weight gain are complex and involve interaction between life-style factors and ADRs. The cause of the weight gain will have to be determined on a balance of probabilities as there is no known single mechanism that adequately explains the weight change seen with antipsychotic medications (Expert Consensus Group 2005).

Obesity and weight gain have long been associated with antipsychotic medications. Silver-stone *et al.* (1988) in a survey of 226 patients attending depot neuroleptic clinics in inner London found the prevalence of clinically relevant obesity was four times that in the general population, suggesting that this has major implications for compliance.

Excess weight and obesity are independent risk factors for a range of chronic physical conditions. The prevalence of obesity among individuals with schizophrenia and affective dis-orders is estimated at 1.5 to 2 times higher than the general population (American Diabetes Association, American Psychiatric Association, American Association of Clinical Endocrin-ologists, North American Association for the Study of Obesity 2004). The effect of this can be seen in the increased prevalence of physical conditions such as diabetes and CHD and higher mortality rates.

Factors that contribute to weight gain

Adverse drug reactions

- Sedation and decreased motivation: clients are too tired to engage in exercise programmes.
- Weight gain is difficult to reverse so it may seem pointless.
- Metabolic disturbances: glucose intolerance and dyslipidaemia increase the risk of obesity.
- Cardiovascular problems: the client may not be able to engage in moderate physical activity.
- Excessive thirst: clients take high calorie drinks that increase weight.
- Problems with balance and gait: these may prevent participation in exercise.

Illness related factors

- Negative symptoms, e.g. decreased motivation may account for a sedentary lifestyle (but this is also a general population factor).
- Clients may withdraw from others due to paranoid ideas.
- Reduced self-esteem: clients may have a poor body image so they are embarrassed to exercise.
- The client may have mania, where the intention is to reduce activity.
- Movement disorders may inhibit potential for exercise.

Other factors

- There may be negative staff attitudes about clients succeeding.
- Social exclusion: clients may not have the resources or support to join gyms and the stigma of mental illness is another barrier.
- There may be a lack of availability of treatment options such as appetite suppressant medica-tion or gastric surgery.

Many of the risk factors for obesity and weight gain are modifiable. Lifestyle advice, healthy eating plans and exercise have all been shown to be valuable in combating obesity and diabetes. Psychotropic medication regimes are also a modifiable risk factor as these can be changed in the face of deteriorating physical health.

Predictors of weight gain

Weight gain is a serious ADR. It is one of the most risky for physical complications but it appears to be grossly underestimated in practice. Predictors for weight gain include

- first episode treatment
- low baseline BMI
- better clinical response
- increased appetite
- high rate of initial weight gain

(The Expert Consensus Group 2005)

When clients are commenced on atypical antipsychotics they should be closely monitored to determine the extent of weight gain. Rettenbacher *et al.* (2006) found that metabolic side effects occur earlier during treatment with atypical antipsychotics, especially olanzapine and clozapine. They found that patients treated with amisulpride or ziprasidone decreased BMI. It would therefore be prudent to commence a weight management programme immediately clients are commenced on atypical medications as this may slow the rate at which weight is gained.

Complications of weight gain

Obese clients are 13 times more likely to request discontinuation of their medication and 3 times more likely to be non-compliant when compared with non-obese clients (Weiden *et al.* 2004, Kurzthaler and Fleischhacker 2001). However, treatment related weight gain may be a marker for clinical improvement in clients (Expert Consensus Group 2005). This irony illustrates that the main factor in selecting medication regimes is effectiveness of treating psychosis. Monitoring weight gain needs to be targeted to be effective. Prioritizing clients will be important and factors to consider include

- clients taking olanzapine and clozapine;
- clients taking psychotropic medication who have other metabolic and lifestyle risk factors;
- clients taking more than one psychotropic medication;
- clients with a family history of obesity, diabetes, stroke or CHD;
- clients taking antipsychotic medication for the first time;
- clients changing from typical to atypical antipsychotics.

Managing weight gain as an ADR

Weiden *et al.* (2004) showed that obese clients are a high risk for stopping medication. Weight gain is not an aesthetic side effect; it is a very serious issue. The health risks related to it are significant and include hypertension, T2D, obesity, CHD and stroke. These need to be considered more seriously.

Managing weight gain will require focus as clients may be at different treatment stages:

- newly diagnosed and treatment naive
- taking psychotropic medication and without weight gain
- taking psychotropic medication with weight gain
- switching from typical to atypical medications

The aim of weight management for some will be to reduce weight gain through health promotion advice, lifestyle changes and possibly a change in medication. For others practitioners should focus on preventing initial weight gain and obesity because subsequent weight loss is very difficult to achieve. The type and severity of metabolic ADRs will also influence their management. Clinicians should focus on preventing weight gain as subsequent weight loss is difficult to achieve and this may lead to demotivation and feelings of failure. Interventions may include

- closer weight monitoring
- engagement in a weight management programme
- use of an adjunctive treatment to reduce weight or manage a co-morbid physical illness
- switching the medication to one with less weight gain liability (NICE 2002)
- clients who suffer from hyper-obesity should be considered for the use of radical responses such as appetite suppressants and/or surgery

An inter-professional approach to managing weight gain is required including a dietician, mental health pharmacist and an exercise therapist or activities nurse who will be able to help plan activities and exercises for the clients. Factors that should be considered for monitoring metabolic ADRs include indicators such as

- BMI
- waist-hip ratio/circumference
- cardiovascular assessment – BP for hypertension, blood lipids for high cholesterol
- diabetes/metabolic syndrome markers
- urinalysis

You will need to prioritize timescales for measuring these indicators. For example, you do not need a weekly waist circumference, urinalysis or monthly blood lipid level. However, short interval BMI, e.g. every three weeks, may initially be required to monitor rapid weight gain. Frequency will depend on individual circumstances. Intervals should be

- baseline
- monthly
- quarterly/six monthly and
- yearly

While monitoring should be targeted it should not be biased. Citrome *et al.* (2003) found that those taking atypical medications were more likely to have glucose screening than those taking typical medications. This presents a clear problem when trying to compare both sets of medications for prevalence of diabetes and may indicate an inequality in health for our clients.

Cardiac system adverse effects

Our clients are at risk of cardiovascular illness due to lifestyle factors, ADRs or a combination of both. Medications such as antipsychotics, e.g. thioridazine, sertindole, ziprasidone and tricyclic antidepressants can cause arrhythmias. Severe cardiac reactions, such as arrhythmias and sudden death have led to the withdrawal of sertindole (Appleby *et al.* 2000). Most classes of drug used in psychiatry affect the cardiac system. It is important that practitioners have skills in assessing cardiovascular health and knowledge of their client's medication regimes (see Chapter 5).

Cardiac side effects are common in psychotropic medication and these can either be minor or severe. Although fatal events have been reported these are not common experiences. Cardiac reactions include

- orthostatic (postural) hypotension
- hypertension
- tachycardia
- cardiac arrhythmias, e.g. ventricular fibrillation

- myocarditis
- pulmonary embolism
- blood dyscrasias

Box 8.4   Specifically, outline the composition of the blood.
Exercise

Disorders of cardiac conduction

Psychotropic medication is associated with changes to the electrical activity of the heart that can lead to fatal cardiac arrhythmias. These changes will be picked up on ECG readings, which is why an ECG should be undertaken under the following circumstances:

- on the commencement of high risk medications
- when changing regimes
- when giving high risk medications to clients with metabolic risk factors
- when giving high risk medications to clients with diagnosed heart conditions
- poly-pharmacy
- following rapid tranquillisation

Electrical activity of the heart

In a normal ECG there are three waves, symbolizing a heart beat (see Chapter 5). The P wave represents atrial depolarization; the QRS wave represents rapid ventricular depolarization; and the T wave indicates ventricular repolarization (Tortora and Derrickson 2006). See Figure 8.1 for a representation of the electrical activity of a normal heart beat. When these waves are occurring in harmony we have a normal cardiac cycle. The average QT interval is 400msec in healthy adults (Marder *et al.* 2004) and a QT interval of 500msec or greater is considered a risk factor sudden death. When these waves are disharmonious – either too quick (tachycardia) or too slow (bradycardia) – then we have an abnormal cardiac cycle. This is referred to as cardiac arrhythmia.

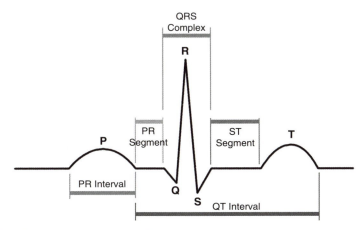

Figure 8.1 The electrical activity of a normal heart beat

Psychotropic medications such as thioridazine (although not commonly used now), sertindole, ziprasidone, olanzapine, quetiapine and tricyclic antidepressants can either prolong the QT or QRS intervals. This leads to cardiac arrhythmias that cause the heart to beat abnormally. In some cases these arrhythmias are serious and can be fatal. These drugs are associated with QT prolongation.

QT prolongation

Psychotropic medication can alter the different waves in the ECG, especially the QT interval (see Figure 8.1). The QT interval represents the time required for completion of both ventricular depolarization and repolarization (Pallavi *et al.* 2004). QT prolongation is a risk factor for ventricular arrhythmia. This may be minor where clients experience palpitations, or it can be serious where a condition called 'torsade de pointes' develops (see Figure 8.2). This is a malignant ventricular arrhythmia that is associated with syncope and sudden death (Glassman and Bigger 2001). O'Brien and Oyebode (2003) state it is associated with non-specific symptoms such as palpitations, dizziness, syncope (fainting) and seizures.

Although a rare ADR it is important to be aware of it and of potential risk factors:

- medications most associated with it;
- the cardiac health/history of clients taking these medications; and
- the presence of other cardiac risk factors.

Psychiatric medications that provoke QT prolongation include antipsychotics (both typical and atypical) and tricyclic antidepressants.

If a client faints as the result of a cardiac event, there is also the danger of a head injury. Practitioners should be extra vigilant with observing clients taking medications that can cause syncope or orthostatic hypotension. You should encourage clients to report any feelings of dizziness, light headedness or changes in consciousness so that they can be investigated.

QRS prolongation

The QRS wave is associated with ventricular depolarization. As the heart tissue of the ventricles is thick (to aid pumping) the passage of the QRS impulse is naturally slightly longer. However, QRS prolongation occurs when the electrical impulse between the atria and the ventricles is impaired. This can lead to heart block where there are dropped heart beats. On an ECG this is represented by the P wave not being followed by the QRS wave.

Changes in duration, structure and amplitude of the ECG waves are diagnostic indicators of cardiac problems which require further investigation. An ECG should be performed at least twice yearly – one to give a baseline reading and another to monitor progress. Clients with cardiac problems taking psychotropic medications may require more frequent ECGs.

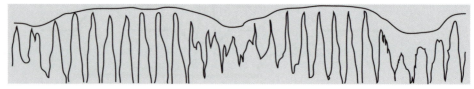

Figure 8.2 ECG representation of torsade de pointes

Myocarditis

Myocarditis is an inflammation of the myocardium that usually occurs as a complication of a viral infection, rheumatic fever or exposure to certain chemicals or medications (Tortora and Derrickson 2006). Research by Killian *et al.* (1999) indicates a risk of fatal myocarditis in patients who take clozapine. Marder *et al.* (2004) found 80 per cent of cases of myocarditis occurred within six weeks of treatment commencing and the mortality rate was 40 per cent. Thirty cases with eight fatalities among 24,108 patients were reported in the UK (Marder *et al.* 2004). Indeed Novartis (2008) suggests that clozapine is associated with an increased risk of fatal myocarditis, especially during, but not limited to, the first month of therapy.

Recognition and management

Myocarditis is a rare event that may go unrecognized by clinicians. Therefore when clients taking clozapine present with the above symptoms, myocarditis should be considered as a primary cause. This should then be confirmed by emergency pathology blood tests, for example, for increased white cell count (eosinophils) and for the cardiac enzyme troponin (see pathology in Table 8.2). If myocarditis is suspected in anyone taking clozapine, treatment should be promptly discontinued (Novartis 2008) and clients referred to a cardiology specialist for further assessment and treatment.

Pulmonary embolism

When a blood clot forms there is a risk that some of it breaks off and enters the blood stream. If this travels to the heart it may cause a pulmonary embolism. This means the pulmonary artery is obstructed preventing blood reaching the heart. This can lead to heart failure as the heart loses its ability to pump correctly.

Pulmonary embolism and deep vein thrombosis have been reported as ADRs of Clozaril (Novartis 2008). Kozier *et al.* (2008b) outline signs and symptoms of pulmonary embolism as

- Sudden chest pain
- Shortness of breath
- Cyanosis
- Shock
- Tachycardia
- Low blood pressure

Table 8.2 Symptoms and pathology of myocarditis

Symptoms of myocarditis	Pathology of myocarditis
Unexplained fatigue	Increase white blood cell count
Dyspnoea	Eosinophilia (increase in eosinophils)*
Tachypnoea	Increased erythrocyte sedimentation rate
Fever	Increased troponin levels (a cardiac enzyme)*
Chest pain	ECG changes – ST abnormalities and T wave inversion
Palpitations	

* important diagnostic indicators

Source: Marder *et al.* 2004

The blood

Blood makes up about 7 per cent of body weight (Waugh and Grant 2006) with the average human having around 8 pints (5.6 litres). The major functions of the blood include

- regulation and maintenance of body temperature
- communication within the body through carrying hormones
- transporting oxygen and nutrients to cells and tissues
- transporting waste material for removal from the body
- transporting white blood cells to fight infection
- transporting platelets to help wound healing
- regulation and maintenance of body pH

Blood composition

The blood is composed of plasma, different types of cells and other elements. Blood plasma contains salts, plasma proteins, hormones and nutrients. Serum plasma is tested when monitoring the levels of certain psychotropic medication levels in the blood. The blood also contains white and red blood cells and thrombocytes (also known as platelets).

Haemopoiesis

Haemopoiesis is the production of blood cells and platelets and is confined to bone marrow (McFerran 2008). Some lymphocytes are produced in lymphoid tissue (Waugh and Grant 2006). Erythropoiesis is the production of red blood cells. Blood cell production is a lifelong process. Each type of blood cell has a life span. When these cells get older they are replaced by newer ones or new cells are produced in response to a crisis, for example, infection.

Red blood cells

Red blood cells (RBCs) transport oxygen from the lungs to cells and tissues and then return carbon dioxide to the lungs. They are produced in bone marrow. RBCs contain haemoglobin which oxygen binds to, producing oxyhaemoglobin. This binding produces high levels of oxygen in the blood, which is measured by pulse oximetry and arterial blood gas assay.

White blood cells

White blood cells (WBCs) fight infection and are produced in bone marrow and the lymphatic system. There are two main types; granulocytes and agranulocytes. WBCs are motile (they move around) and phagocytic (they ingest germs). There are five different types:

- Neutrophils – prevent and remove bacteria and fungi from entering the body
- Eosinophils – target parasites and promote inflammation in allergic reactions
- Basophils – involved in allergic reactions
- Monocytes – ingest and digest foreign bodies, also involved in antibody production
- Lymphocytes – make antibodies and also destroy foreign bodies

Thrombocytes (platelets)

Platelets are produced in bone marrow and contain a variety of substances that promote blood clotting and stop bleeding (Waugh and Grant 200). This complex process is called haemostasis.

Overproduction of platelets can lead to blood clotting (thrombosis) which is a risk factor for stroke. Underproduction can lead to excessive bleeding where difficulties in forming blood clots occur.

Relevance for mental health nurses

This knowledge is very important as some psychotropic medications cause blood dyscrasias. Dyscrasia is defined as an abnormal state of the body due to abnormal development or metabolism (McFerran 2008). Blood dyscrasias include abnormal production and reduction of all blood cells. This can affect the client's immune system and their ability to fight infection or their ability to heal following a self-inflicted injury.

Blood dyscrasias as ADRs

Table 8.3 shows blood dyscrasias linked to certain medications used in psychiatry. Agranulocytosis is a severe and acute deficiency of neutrophils (white blood cells; McFerran 2008). Neutrophils are a primary defence against infection. Agranulocytosis is potentially very severe which is why clozapine is so strictly monitored. Clients prescribed clozapine must have regular mandatory blood tests to measure their white blood cell count to ensure the immune system is not compromised.

Clozapine monitoring

Theisen *et al.* (2001) note that despite its considerable advantages in treating psychosis, clozapine's value is limited by the potentially life threatening agranulocytosis. Novartis (2008) caution that clients should be prompted to report symptoms of agranulocytosis which include lethargy, weakness, fever and sore throat.

Clients receiving clozapine need to have regular blood monitoring for dyscrasias. White blood cell (WBC) and absolute neutrophil count (ANC) are usually taken before initiation of treatment, weekly for six months, then two weekly for a further six months, then finally four weekly, if results are stable (see Novartis 2008).

Other potential reactions

Clozapine reduces seizure threshold so epileptic seizures are a risk in clients taking larger does. Clients with epilepsy or a history of seizures should be carefully monitored.

Table 8.3 Associated blood dyscrasias as adverse drug reactions

	Leucopenia	Agranulocytosis	Thrombocytopenia	Anaemia	Neutropenia
Medication					
Chlorpromazine	X	X			
Clozapine	X	X[1]		X	X
Olanzapine	X		X		X
Zotepine	X		X	X	
Quetiapine	X				X
Amitriptyline	X	X	X		
Carbamazepine	X	X	X	X[2]	
Phenytoin	X		X	X[3]	

[1]can be fatal, [2]aplastic anaemia, [3]megaloblastic anaemia

Source: Adapted from the British National Formulary 2007

Anaemia

In anaemia there is not enough haemoglobin available to carry sufficient oxygen from the lungs to supply the needs of tissues (Waugh and Grant 2006: 68). This decreases the amount of oxygenated blood which contributes to the following:

- Fatigue – chronic tiredness due to lack of oxygen supply to muscles
- Breathlessness/abnormal respirations – increased respiration as a means of compensation for low oxygen supply
- Hypertension – the heart has to work harder to supply the same amount of oxygen
- Less perfusion of tissues which can lead to tissue death as seen in myocardial infarction
- Low mood – depression may occur as a reaction to reduced social functioning and inability to perform usual tasks

Haemoglobin may be reduced due to a lack of production of RBCs, the presence of immature RBCs that don't have haemoglobin, blood loss or RBCs being destroyed. There are some particular types of anaemia that we should be aware of.

Aplastic anaemia

Aplastic anaemia is a serious condition where the body cannot produce RBCs. In cases such as this a bone marrow transplant is required. Causes of aplastic anaemia are genetic or may occur due to reactions to some medications (see Table 8.3).

Megaloblastic anaemia

Megaloblastic anaemia is caused by a deficiency of vitamin B_{12} or folic acid. This causes RBCs to be immature and deformed. Types of megaloblastic anaemia include:

- *Iron deficiency anaemia*: this is diagnosed when an individual's blood tests are below 9g/dl (Waugh and Grant 2006). Poor diet, which is a risk factor in our client group, is a cause of this.
- *Pernicious anaemia*: this is caused by vitamin B_{12} deficiency. This is an autoimmune disorder which can occur as a result of prolonged alcohol use. Symptoms of pernicious anaemia are physical and neurological. They include fine or coarse tremor, lateral nystagmus, alcohol related dementia and peripheral neuropathy. Management is usually reintroducing vitamin B_{12} either by oral or intra-muscular injection. The intra-muscular injection is an oily substance which can be quite painful for clients to have. You should exercise great care when giving it so that it disperses well and does not go on to form an abscess.

Anaemia due to low blood volume

Following an incident of severe cutting or repeated incidents in a short period, the client may have lost enough blood to render them temporarily anaemic. A full blood count should be considered in such circumstances as symptoms of anaemia may be confused with symptoms of depression following the self-harm incident. Furthermore, depending on the type of implement used there may be a risk of the client developing an infection.

Sickle cell anaemia

Sickle cell anaemia is a haemolytic anaemia and occurs when red blood cells are destroyed prematurely (thalassaemia is another type). This is an inherited blood disorder where abnormal haemoglobin molecules become misshapen when deoxygenated making them sickle shaped (Waugh and Grant 2006). This disorder primarily affects individuals from an African Caribbean background.

Assessment

Anaemia is usually diagnosed by a series of blood tests such as

- Full blood count (FBC)
- Iron (Hb) levels
- Liver function test
- Bone marrow biopsy (in very severe cases)

Treatment

In severe cases a bone marrow transplant is required. In other cases drugs that stimulate RBC production will be prescribed. In the majority of cases iron supplements will be prescribed and changes to the diet that introduce more iron will be made. Treatment of anaemia will depend on the cause and on how far below the normal range the Hb level falls. For example, a small fall might be reversed with dietary changes, a moderate fall with dietary changes and iron supplements and severe falls (e.g. following severe self-harm) in more invasive interventions such as transfusion.

Other blood related effects

SSRI antidepressants can cause bleeding disorders such as ecchymosis and purpura. Ecchymosis is a bluish-black mark, resembling a bruise, on the skin. This results from the release of blood into the tissue either through injury or spontaneous leaking of blood from the vessels (McFerran 2008). Purpura is a condition where red or purple blotches form under the skin as a result of bleeding from small capillaries. This may be caused by thrombocytopenia. These blotches resemble those found as a symptom of meningitis – they do not disappear on blanching. This should be remembered when conducting a physical exam. If you notice these you will need to document it and report it to the doctor for further investigation.

Sexual dysfunction and adverse drug reactions

Prolactin is a hormone produced by the pituitary gland. Its function is to stimulate progesterone and lactation (McFerran 2008). The normal values for prolactin are less than 25mcg/L in females and less than 20mcg/L in males. Breast enlargement and lactation are natural responses in pregnancy. Therefore pregnancy can elevate the levels of prolactin in preparation for childbirth. In pregnant women the normal range of prolactin is 20–400mcg/L.

Dopamine inhibits prolactin release so blocking dopamine receptors will increase the risk of developing sexual dysfunction due to increased levels of prolactin. Hyperprolactinaemia is an excess of the hormone, in the absence of pregnancy, and this is an adverse reaction of psychotropic medication. This can lead to extremely unpleasant side effects in both men and women:

- In men: difficulty in reaching orgasm, reduced libido (desire for sex), ejaculation problems such as impotence or premature ejaculation. Gynaecomastia (development of breasts) may also occur;
- In women: symptoms that mimic pregnancy such as amenorrhoea – the absence of the

period – or disruption of the menstrual cycle, reduced libido, reduced bone density and osteoperosis;
- In both: galactorrhoea, which is abnormal breast milk production.

Most types of psychotropic medications act on dopamine receptors and therefore cause problems with sexual function. Antipsychotic medications, particularly risperidone, can cause hyperprolactinaemia (Jones and Jones 2008). SSRIs, typical and atypical antipsychotics and lithium can elevate prolactin levels.

Priapism

Priapism is a painful condition where clients experience an erection in the absence of any stimulus. A significant problem is that the erection can last for hours. This can be a distressing and embarrassing experience for the client. Mostly it is very painful. Treating priapism involves aspirating blood from the penis (about 20–50ml; BNF 2007). This reduces the erection. Given the nature of the treatment it may need to be done in an accident and emergency or acute hospital environment. Clients should be accompanied by someone they are familiar with, who knows the problem and who the client feels can offer them support and reassurance.

If the procedure is undertaken in a mental health unit it will need to be a sterile procedure following the principles of aseptic technique, promoting infection control and controlled disposal of clinical waste products. Needless to say, clients will be very distressed and you will need to explain the procedure in language they understand, offering continual reassurance and support throughout.

Physical investigations, antipsychotic medications and adverse drug reactions

> **Box 8.5**   Which adverse drug reaction would you rather have – tardive dyskinesia or obesity?
> **Exercise**   Why?

Atypical antipsychotics are the recognized first line treatment for schizophrenia in the UK (NICE 2002). Practitioners should focus on developing good practice in monitoring ADRs due to the increased risk of higher morbidity and mortality in our clients. However, which tools are there to use or which guidance can we look to? These are common questions, with no clear answers. There is a general lack of consensus as to what to monitor and when and even who should do the monitoring – primary or secondary care services, doctors or nurses.

Adverse drug reactions are normally measured using checklists such as the Abnormal Involuntary Movement Scale (AIMS; Guy 1976), the Side-Effect Scale/Checklist for Antipsychotic Medication (SESCAM; Bennett et al. 1995), or the Liverpool University Neuroleptic Side-effect Rating Scale (LUNSERS; Day et al. 1995). These scales are generally in the tradition of abnormal movements, sedation and Parkinsonian type symptoms. Jordan et al. (2004) compared different rating scales for the parameters of ADRs assessed and found little focus on 'physical' side effects. For example, orthostatic hypotension is a known effect of psychotropic medication yet only one of the six rating scales examined had both a sitting and standing blood pressure assessment.

The LUNSERS (Day et al. 1995) includes ten questions referred to as 'red herrings' – imaginary reactions such as mouth ulcers or runny nose to screen over-reporters. However, Jordan et al.

(2004) suggest that far from being imaginary, mouth ulcers could arise from xerostomia and runny nose from alpha blockade induced by antipsychotics. It may be a symptom of the lack of regard for physical health that there is a lack of rating scales, or that rating scales tend to exclude physical ADRs. At worst they may inadvertently promote diagnostic overshadowing through minimizing a client's experiences and not interpreting them as credible symptoms.

There are some baseline indicators that can help to inform good practice and these should be client centred. Figure 8.3 indicates factors for physical health monitoring that need to be considered for:

- clients who will be taking medication for the first time where baseline measurements will allow for comparison with future screening;
- clients who have been established on medication and who may not have had their physical health monitored, so there is no credible baseline for comparison;
- clients taking more than one psychotropic medication. The important difference between all three groups will be in interventions for physical health. In new clients assessment may lead to primary prevention, e.g. of weight gain, where as in established clients it may be secondary or tertiary interventions to reduce weight gain. Nevertheless some type of protocol will need to be established at a local level.

Timescales

How often should these investigations occur? Again there is no real consensus. If money were no object then very routinely. However, to utilize resources effectively investigations need to be targeted. The inter-professional team should decide on timescales using guidance by pharmaceutical companies, best practice guidelines (e.g. NICE), observations from practitioners and self-reporting of clients/carers.

Two timeframes are required: at baseline and at one year. This will give two results to

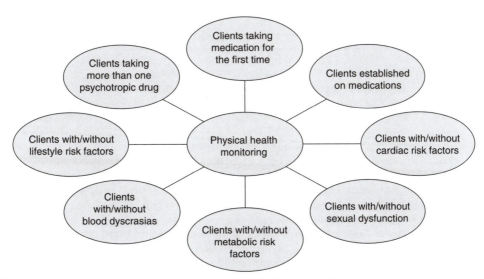

Figure 8.3 Factors to consider when monitoring physical effects of medication

compare everything with. In between times other investigations may be carried out more routinely than others, e.g. at every contact baseline observations can be taken. The results of these may prompt further investigation, for example, unstable blood pressure for four consecutive readings may lead to an ECG.

Prioritizing may begin with those who have a physical illness or increased risk that requires greater monitoring. Some timeframes are set by the nature of the treatment regime, e.g. monitoring WBCs and lithium levels for clozapine and lithium respectively. With regard to lithium, NICE (2006a) recommends an annual physical health review, normally in primary care, to assess for clients with bipolar disorder:

- lipid levels, including cholesterol in all patients over 40 even if there is no other indication of risk;
- plasma glucose levels;
- weight;
- smoking status and alcohol use;
- blood pressure.

This latter approach monitors physical health from a specific illness perspective. NICE (2006a) recommends the following approach for clients taking antipsychotics.

- Weight checked every 3 months for the first year, and more often if they gain weight rapidly;
- Plasma glucose and lipids (preferably fasting levels) should be measured 3 months after the start of treatment (and within 1 month if taking olanzapine), and more often if there is evidence of elevated levels;
- In patients taking risperidone, prolactin levels should be measured if symptoms of raised prolactin develop; these include low libido, sexual dysfunction, menstrual abnormalities, gynaecomastia and galactorrhoea.

Monitoring may also be required in clients with physical conditions following a critical event such as rapid tranquillization where poly-pharmacy may be required. While it is impossible to cover all eventualities in monitoring ADRs some areas that practitioners should consider for physical monitoring for psychotropic medications are outlined in Table 8.4.

Improving concordance and health education

Box 8.6 Exercise	What is your role in promoting compliance with medication?

Psychotropic medications have always been associated with variable compliance, even when clinical improvements have been evident. ADRs are a key cause of non-compliance. Clients are the only ones that can suffer from these and practitioners must cope with the fallout from this. Non-compliance and partial compliance with medication in people with schizophrenia is estimated at one third respectively (Oehl *et al.* 2000). This means only one third of clients comply with their medication.

In a survey of American clients Weiden *et al.* (2004) found that higher BMI and subjective distress from weight gain were predictors of non-compliance. Obese individuals were more than twice as likely as those with a normal BMI to report missing their medication. Tschoner *et al.* (2007: 1356) state that according to patients, psychosocial consequences of weight gain, such as a sense of demoralization, physical discomfort and being the target of sustained social

Table 8.4 Areas practitioners should consider for physical monitoring for psychotropic medications

Aspect	Clinical investigation/measurement	Rationale
Client physical history	Cardiovascular illness Respiratory disease Diabetes Any other medical or surgical history	To get a baseline of current physical health issues so that medication regimes can reflect any risk issues
Lifestyle risk factors	Current diet (estimated calories) Smoking Substance misuse Physical activity	Smoking, alcohol use, illicit substance use and caffeine use are risk factors in cardiovascular illness Low levels of physical activity and poor diet lead to obesity
Client family history	Cardiovascular illness and stroke Obesity Diabetes	Family history might present with a genetic predisposition for physical illness
Clinical observations	Blood pressure Pulse ECG Body mass index Waist measurement Waist-hip ratio Urinalysis	To determine cardiac function and to assess weight gain which is a risk factor in cardiovascular illness ECG is important as QT readings greater than 450msecs will need careful cardiac assessment, greater than 500msecs may mean prescribing another medication Urinalysis will screen for metabolic and other problems
Blood tests	Sodium and potassium levels, cholesterol levels, Fasting blood sugar (FBS) Cardiac enzymes, White blood cells Liver function test Renal function Thyroid function test Prolactin levels	Psychotropic medications can affect potassium concentration that can lead to QT prolongation High cholesterol is a risk factor for atherosclerosis FBS to screen for T2D In clozapine, Troponin for suspected risk of myocarditis White blood cell count should be done to exclude neutropenia Renal and thyroid function is recommended for clients on long term lithium therapy

stigma are so intolerable that they may discontinue treatment even if it is effective. Kurzthaler and Fleischhacker (2001) found that weight gain was a risk factor for non-compliance, reduced quality of life and social retreat, i.e. clients not wanting to socialize.

It is evident that weight gain influences compliance. However, in a small study exploring clients' and clinicians' concerns about side effects Huffman *et al.* (2004) found that clients ranked cognitive slowing as more adverse while mental health nurses rated weight gain as more adverse than clients or psychiatrists. A reason for this is that clients may not have had health promotion interventions regarding the importance of lifestyle factors or weight gain as a severe reaction.

The following indicates an example of the process that practitioners should use when they are discussing medications with clients:

1 Discuss the potential benefits
2 Discuss the potential adverse reactions
3 Perform a physical health check for baseline readings
4 Record weight and body mass index
5 Record smoking behaviour
6 Assess alcohol intake
7 Advise not to stop medication without first discussing it
8 Encourage to disclose if they have stopped medication

In practice, however, many people are not told about possible adverse reactions.

Ethical issues

Practitioners need to think very carefully about the implications of caring for clients taking medications that are associated with increased mortality and morbidity. Möller (2000) suggests that atypical antipsychotics will be better accepted by clients because fewer side effects will lead to increased compliance providing a better quality of life. This is a standard defence in the use of atypical medications – fewer means better. However, fewer does not necessarily mean less severe. The only true judge of the adverse drug reactions is the client who will probably continue to experience them for as long as they take them.

Practitioners, especially nurse prescribers, must fully appreciate the ethical aspects of clients taking medication that has the potential to leave them with a chronic physical condition, or worse. While it is good practice to highlight the positive aspects of medication on mental health, practitioners must step up to the challenge of physical adverse drug reactions. One cannot shrug off 10kg of weight gain with an observation that 'at least your voices are gone'. Weight gain can affect self-esteem, lead to increased social exclusion and compromise physical health.

Conclusion

Although rare, adverse drug reactions can sometimes be fatal. We need to have the prerequisite knowledge and skills to assess and screen for physical ADRs in order to reduce any risks to the client. This is one reason why we need to have good knowledge of physical care. We must also be diligent with our physical assessment as Reilly et al. (2002) found that information on smoking, drinking or taking illicit drugs was usually missing from the patient case notes.

Summary of key points

- Practitioners are required to have the skills and knowledge in recognizing adverse drug reactions.
- Practitioners should use guidelines for physical screening of clients taking various psychotropic medications.
- Practitioners should implement recommendations regarding monitoring physical health in clients taking medication from expert groups, e.g. NICE.
- Practitioners should keep up to date with adverse drug reactions when clients commence new types of medications or change medication regimes.

Quick quiz

1 List five common physical adverse drug reactions that may be experienced by clients taking typical antipsychotics.
2 List five common physical adverse drug reactions that may be experienced by clients taking atypical antipsychotics.
3 What is the therapeutic serum plasma level for someone taking lithium?
4 What effects are associated with increased prolactin levels?
5 What is a normal blood cholesterol level?

9 | Physical health emergencies in mental health settings

By the end of this chapter you will be able to:

- Identify specific medical emergencies in mental health settings
- Recognize risk factors that can contribute to medical emergencies
- Understand the role of the mental health nurse in various medical emergencies
- Identify how the nurse can provide care to clients in a state of collapse
- Describe the nursing care priorities during medical emergency

Box 9.1
Exercise What are the basic principles of life support?

Introduction

In 2007a NICE published clinical guidelines for acutely ill patients in hospital. Although the emphasis is on acute hospital settings there are some very good pointers that can be utilized in mental health settings. These guidelines emphasize that the sooner we recognize physical deterioration and intervene, the better the outcomes are for the client.

Early detection is based on 'track and trigger' systems. Physiological track and trigger systems rely on periodic observation of selected basic physiological signs ('tracking') with predetermined calling or response criteria ('trigger') for requesting the attendance of staff who have specific competencies in the management of acute illness and/or critical care (NICE 2007a). For example, baseline observations and blood serum levels may be track and trigger criteria for lithium toxicity.

Professional responsibilities regarding clinical observations must be clear. For students this will be competence in taking, recording and passing on information regarding the physical observations and for qualified practitioners it will be competence in acting on the readings. NICE (2007a) recommends that staff caring for patients in acute hospital settings should have competencies in monitoring, measurement, interpretation and prompt response to the acutely ill patient appropriate to the level of care they are providing.

The National Patient Safety Agency (2008) revealed wide variations in standards of resuscitation in mental health and learning disability settings. Of 599 reports of at least moderate harm related to choking or cardiac/respiratory arrest, they found 26 incidents of significant lack of staff knowledge or skills, for example, in identifying cardiac arrest or of equipment availability, e.g. basic mask-to-mouth devices. Needless to say we all have a professional duty to be up to date with our first aid or basic life support training.

Emergency medical equipment

Metherall *et al.* (2006) set up twenty-four-hour medical emergency response teams (MERTs) to ensure effective responses to medical and psychiatric emergencies. Each MERT has an emergency bag that contains the following equipment with other equipment brought from wards as required:

- Pulse oximeter
- Thermometer
- Manual sphygmomanometer and stethoscope
- Blood glucose monitoring machine
- Pocket face mask
- Selection of guedal airways
- Variety of first aid equipment including gloves and gauze
- Tuff cut shears
- Ligature cutters
- Pen torch
- Paperwork – pen, dry wipe pen, log book, pre-arrest call criteria, record of cardiac arrest form and physical observations chart

Other equipment that should be on standby includes

- Suction machine
- Defibrillator
- Emergency trolley

What do we mean by medical emergencies in mental health?

A medical emergency is any event that poses a serious risk to the physical health of a client. This risk is normally immediate, e.g. myocardial infarction. However, it can also be gradual, unless immediate care is given to reduce the risk, e.g. minor lithium toxicity if left undetected and untreated will develop into an immediate emergency. Physical assessment skills will allow practitioners to determine if the event they are assessing is of a routine or emergency nature. We explore the following medical emergencies explored in this:

- cardiac arrest
- respiratory arrest
- ECT and post-general anaesthetic recovery
- diabetic emergencies – hyperglycaemia, diabetic ketoacidosis and hypoglycaemia
- haemorrhage
- overdose
- intoxication
- lithium toxicity
- neuroleptic malignant syndrome
- serotonin syndrome
- rapid tranquillization

Responses to medical emergencies are crucial for the client's immediate and long term health.

If medical or nursing care is not given immediately it may result in a poor outcome. If interventions are not sustained this may also negatively impact on the client's outcomes. Responses to medical emergencies need to be swift and coordinated and you should know the medical emergency policy of your workplace.

The primary aim of intervention in a medical emergency is to prevent further deterioration of physical health in areas of respiration and circulation; this may be achieved by

- Basic first aid
- Basic and/or advanced life support
- Medical interventions including
  - Defibrillation
  - Intubation
  - Giving emergency medications, e.g. adrenaline
- Immediate transfer to an intensive care facility

The outcome of any intervention is not guaranteed but all possible interventions should be given and maintained until such a time as the client is either recovered; transferred to an appropriate medical facility; or pronounced dead by a doctor.

Basic principles of first aid and basic life support

As nurses we do not receive certification as first aiders as part of our training, even though our training covers principles of first aid. We may be offered the opportunity to become designated first aiders as part of our in-house training, but this seems a ridiculous irony. Whatever the local policy regarding first aid is, we should all have attended a course on basic life support (BLS). BLS is regarded as a mandatory training requirement for all staff as are the refresher/updates. If you have not completed such a course you should do so as a matter of urgency.

BLS may be required when we find a client in a state of collapse and is a combination of rescue breathing (mouth to mouth) and chest compressions performed to preserve life. This combination sustains some form of cardio-respiratory activity which can keep a person alive until emergency services arrive. Most mental health units will have a defibrillation machine which should be used as part of life support. These are relatively straightforward to use and instruction in how to use one will be a feature of the aforementioned training.

On discovering someone unconscious a primary survey is conducted and consists of checking the response of the casualty:

- **A** – Airway: opening the airway
- **B** – Breathing: checking for breathing
- **C** – Circulation: observing any major bleeding

(Kindleysides 2007)

A secondary survey is conducted if the client is alert. This includes checking each part of the body from head to toe to assess the extent of any injury or illness and following this treatment can be given (Kindleysides 2007).

What might cause collapse?

There are many avenues to collapse and the better we know our clients and their medical backgrounds then the better informed we will be regarding causes of any collapse. Depending on the severity, the medical emergencies listed on p. 175 may have collapse as a feature.

Cardiac arrest

Cardiac arrest occurs when the heart suddenly stops. This prevents the flow of oxygenated blood to the vital organs. It is a medical emergency requiring prompt intervention. Following the primary survey you need to begin chest compressions and rescue breathing. In the UK the recommended ratio is 30 chest compressions for 2 rescue breaths (Resuscitation Council UK 2005). The algorithm shown in Figure 9.1 is usually used in UK hospitals. For community practitioners who find a client collapsed at home a 999 call should be used and neighbours can also be called to help. BLS would commence until paramedics arrive.

**Box 9.2
Exercise**   What are the signs and symptoms of cardiac arrest?

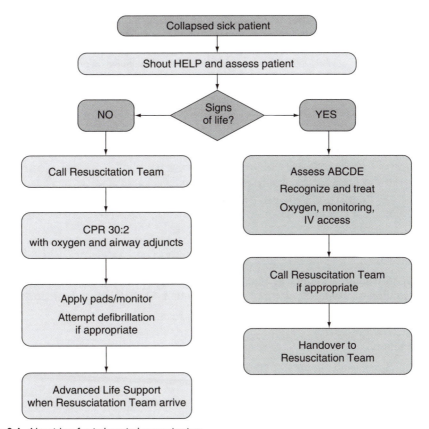

Figure 9.1 Algorithm for in hospital resuscitation

Source: Resuscitation Council UK (2005) reproduced with permission from the Resuscitation Council UK

Box 9.3 Case example

Kwame is a 50-year-old male with a history of psychotic disorder and hypertension. His current medication is chlorpromazine 100mg QID and procyclidine 5mg BD. He smokes 40 cigarettes daily, takes little exercise and eats an irregular and unhealthy diet. Janet finds Kwame in a state of collapse in the bathroom. What does Janet do?

1 Janet tries to rouse Kwame by calling his name and gently shaking him: Kwame remains unresponsive.
2 Janet monitors A, B, C.
3 Janet shouts for help and pulls the emergency alarm cord in the bathroom area. Kwame does not have a pulse, he is cold and clammy to touch and is not breathing.
4 Janet begins to give basic life support – 30 chest compressions followed by two rescue breaths (the first two rescue breaths are not necessary; Resuscitation Council UK 2005).
5 Help arrives and Janet tells them Kwame has had a cardiac arrest. Janet instructs one nurse to get the pulse oximeter and defibrillator and the other to call in a medical emergency. The defibrillator arrives and Janet proceeds to administer advanced life support. She then attaches the pulse oximeter.
6 The duty doctor and crash team arrive, Janet quickly hands over and leaves Kwame in their care.

Janet's diagnosis is cardiac arrest. This is based on her knowledge of

• physical health
• Kwame's history and condition
• her BLS training

Her actions are swift and coordinated and in line with established practice. This is the level of practice required for effective interventions in a medical emergency situation.

Respiratory arrest

Respiratory failure is defined as inadequate gas exchange – hypoxaemia – where there is reduced oxygenation of arterial blood (Brashers and Huether 2004). Signs of respiratory failure include

• No discernable respirations
• Unconsciousness
• Cyanosis

In respiratory arrest clients stop breathing due to

• Airway obstruction e.g. asphyxiation
• Drug overdose
• Injury or trauma
• Prelude to cardiac arrest

In mental health settings respiratory arrest may be caused by asphyxiation, e.g. hanging or suffocation with car fumes. It is important that action is prompt and direct. The client may still have a pulse so the main priority is to recommence breathing either by rescue breathing or mechanically. The principles of the primary survey and the resuscitation algorithm in Figure 8.4 will be used. If you discover someone hanging you should

- Call for help
- Cut the person down, but be careful that they do not fall and sustain a head injury
- Remove the ligature
- Initiate BLS
- Transfer to a medical setting

You should try to stabilize the client's head during the BLS as we do not want to induce further trauma to the neck area. You should also observe the client in case they vomit, carefully placing them in the recovery position to prevent choking. Suction, oxygen and pulse oximetry equipment should be available. BLS will be employed and respirations monitored until the emergency team arrives and the client's care is transferred to them.

Risks to physical health during restraint

Clients may suffer respiratory arrest or other physical injury during physical restraint (see Table 9.1). Prior to physical restraint, the team directly involved should consider the following in all cases, but especially where there is a known history of cardiac illness:

- Know the client's physical history.
- Know the client's medications and how these might increase any risks.
- Follow good practice guidance on the use of physical restraint, e.g. NICE Guidelines (2005).
- Know the medical emergency policy.

During restraint signs such as skin colour, breathing and posture should be noted. Pulse oximetry should also be used especially post-intervention. Post-restraint care includes observation of vital signs, respiratory assessment, observation for cyanosis and possibly ECG.

The following equipment should be available so that a rapid response can be initiated in the event of a medical emergency (NICE 2005):

- suction machine
- defibrillator
- first-line resuscitation medications
- a bag valve mask
- cannulas and fluids
- oxygen

ECT and post-general anaesthetic recovery

ECT is a controversial treatment in mental health. In ECT clients receive a general anaesthetic so it is important that 'ECT nurses' are trained in post-operative recovery techniques, respiratory

Table 9.1 Potential injuries arising from physical restraint

Potential injury	Description
Hypoxia	A lack of oxygen in the blood which affects the heart and other organs. This can arise following respiratory arrest due to postural asphyxiation.
Adverse drug reaction	Neuroleptic malignant syndrome, cardiac arrest
Physical injury	Muscle, skin, bone injury
Risk related to rapid tranquillization	Needlestick injury – to both client and practitioner Risk of infection if a blood spillage

assessment and advanced life support, even though a qualified anaesthetist and doctor will be part of the ECT team. Cullen (2004) suggests that the ECT nurse should have knowledge of

- the actions required in the event of a medical emergency (e.g. suxamethonium apnoea, malignant hyperpyrexia, laryngospasm);
- the drugs used for ECT, their appropriate doses, potential side effects and the appropriate treatment of these;
- dosing policy;
- the local protocol for termination of prolonged seizures.

Nursing care prior to ECT

ECT involves administration of a general anaesthetic so the client should be fasted for 8–10 hours prior to the procedure (check your local policy as fasting times may be different). Medication is generally not given prior to ECT; however, if a client has an existing condition they may be permitted it. The client should be encouraged to go to the toilet prior to treatment to prevent soiling of clothes. Once in the ECT area the nurse will ask the client to remove any objects that may cause harm during the seizure; this includes dentures, prostheses, jewellery and nail varnish (Patton 2008).

Nursing care following ECT should be as follows:

- The recovery area must contain suction, monitoring and emergency equipment.
- Oxygen should be administered routinely to the patient.
- Maintain the client's airway and regularly monitor/record vital signs.
- The client should be observed by a staff member until they wake up.
- When ready the client should be escorted to a final stage area for refreshments and rest until the recovery staff deem them fit to return to the ward.
- The recovery nurse should pass on information to the ward nurse/escort about the client's condition, medication administered, behaviour, untoward procedures or treatment response.
- The client should be encouraged to rest.
- If the client complains of a headache or muscle soreness, analgesia such as paracetamol may be administered.
- Nausea may be treated with an anti-emetic.
- Ward staff should continue to provide support to the client.

(adapted from Finch 2005)

Box 9.4   What are the signs and symptoms of hypoglycaemia?
Exercise

Diabetic emergencies

Homeostasis of glucose control

In a state of homeostasis we have a balance between blood glucose and insulin levels. An imbalance can lead to too much glucose in our system (hyperglycaemia) or too little glucose (hypoglycaemia). When glucose levels increase beta cells in the pancreas are stimulated to release insulin, which acts to lower blood glucose levels. When glucose levels decrease glucagon is released prompting the liver to break down stores of glycogen, which raises blood glucose levels. Hyperglycaemia and hypoglycaemia are two emergencies that we can encounter in mental health settings.

Hyperglycaemia

In Chapter 8 we explored metabolic adverse drug reactions and examined how atypical anti-psychotics seem to have a greater propensity for these. Hyperglycaemia can result in new-onset T2D, metabolic acidosis or ketosis, and even hyperglycaemia related deaths (Llorente and Urrutia 2006). Hyperglycaemia can occur when

- the body does not produce enough insulin;
- the client has not taken their insulin;
- the client has under-dosed, e.g. due to poor injection technique;
- insulin therapy regime is not adequate;
- the client has eaten too much sugary or starchy food;
- the client has a physical illness such as an infection.

If left untreated hyperglycaemia can lead to diabetic ketoacidosis (DKA) which is a potentially life-threatening condition where blood glucose levels become extremely high. Provan (2007) suggests that DKA should be considered as a diagnosis in unconscious or hyperventilating clients. Symptoms may include:

- nausea/vomiting
- polyuria
- polydipsia
- fatigue
- stiff or aching muscles
- weak, rapid pulse
- 'pear drop' breath
- Kussmaul breathing
- confusion or clouding of consciousness
- abdominal cramps

If left untreated the person can fall into a diabetic coma and die.

Clinical investigations that can be used to diagnose DKA include

- Blood tests – a blood glucose level greater than 12mmol/l (Palmer 2004)
- Metabolic acidosis – pH <7.53 (measured in arterial blood gases)
- Pulse oximetry for oxygen saturation
- Urinalysis indicating high readings for ketones and glucose
- Tachycardia
- Hyperpnoea

Nursing intervention in diabetic ketoacidosis

If any clients have diabetes mellitus then you should be aware of the potential complications of hyperglycaemia. Diabetic ketoacidosis (DKA) is a complication that requires prompt intervention. You should ask your client routine questions as a means of eliciting information about their condition, for example, have you lost consciousness, or experienced changes in your level of consciousness, e.g. confusion or unusual sleepiness?

DKA is a medical emergency and immediate medical help is required if you notice any signs or symptoms. If you are not sure of the dosage of insulin or whether the client has taken insulin, then do not attempt to administer insulin. Wait for emergency help. Palmer (2004) suggests that we use the first seven letters of the alphabet as a guide to intervention in DKA:

- A – Airway support – depending on level of consciousness
- B – Breathing – administer oxygen and monitor respiratory rate and rhythm
- C – Circulation – monitor blood pressure and pulse
- D – Drug therapy – insulin will be required as part of the emergency treatment
- E – Electrolyte replacement – an IV infusion may be required to replace sodium and potassium lost during polyuria and/or vomiting
- F – Fluid resuscitation – to correct dehydration
- G – Gases – monitor arterial blood gases for metabolic acidosis

It is important that you have some training in the area of diabetes and DKA. Assessing training needs is explored in the next chapter.

Hypoglycaemia

When there is insufficient glucose in circulation hypoglycaemia can occur. This can be due to

- insulin overdose (purposive or accidental)
- inadequate dietary intake
- missed meals
- excessive exercise
- alcohol use

Signs of hypoglycaemia include (Huether and McCance 2004):

- fatigue
- pallor
- hunger
- confusion
- sweating
- palpitations
- tachycardia
- restlessness
- tremors
- headache

Without treatment, convulsions, coma and death may follow.

In the early stages of hypoglycaemia clients will experience sweating, hand tremor, hunger and palpitations. These should be used as early warning signs when we educate clients in maintaining their health. At this stage a sweet drink or a high sugar snack should restore glucose balance.

If your client experiences changes in consciousness refer to the ward doctor or GP. If you find a client in a state of collapse then summon emergency help and give BLS as required, e.g. place the client in the recovery position. All wards should have an emergency injection of glucagon which should be used in unconscious clients as giving oral agents might lead to choking. You should not attempt to administer insulin. Once glucagon has been administered the client should regain consciousness. You should talk to them and give reassurance. They should be examined by the doctor and regular observations undertaken.

Haemorrhage

In mental health settings clients who self harm by cutting are at risk of losing blood. A severe cut can lead to significant blood loss which can cause hypovolaemia – decreased blood volume in circulation (see Table 9.2). Hypovolaemia increases the risk of shock and cardiac arrest due to the decreased supply of blood and the increased strain being placed on the heart to pump blood more quickly to vital organs and tissue. Prompt action to stem bleeding and transfer to an emergency setting is a priority.

Discovering someone who has cut themselves severely can be a frightening and distressing experience, for both client and staff. Nurses should be calm and professional when they are dealing with such incidents and should not be judgemental. Our first priority is their physical well-being.

If the client is unconscious and bleeding then this is a medical emergency. An ambulance should be called for and the client supported with BLS. They should be placed in the recovery position and pressure applied to the wound to stem the bleeding. Be careful to ensure that the implement used in the incident is not embedded in the wound as applying pressure to this can result in further injury.

You should also remember the principles of infection control and use appropriate barrier methods when providing care, e.g. gloves and an apron. Implements used in the incident should be disposed of in a sharps box. Following the incident it is important that the area is sanitized and all hazardous waste appropriately disposed of.

For the conscious client wound location should be assessed. For example, if the site of cutting is the neck area you may have to maintain an open airway as blood may cause an obstruction. For arm or leg wounds you will have to stem the flow of bleeding. Gauze should be applied directly over the wound and firm pressure placed on this. Limbs should be raised above heart level to reduce blood loss, e.g. for leg wounds clients should be prone and their leg elevated. Clients should not eat or drink anything at this stage and you should continuously monitor their breathing and level of consciousness. Reassurance should be given while waiting for transfer to an acute hospital setting.

Overdose

Overdose can be a curious event in mental health. Sometimes the client may come and tell you they have taken something or they may say nothing and be found in a state of collapse. The

Table 9.2 Effects of blood or fluid loss

Approximate fluid lost	Effects on the body
0.5 litre (about one pint)	Very little or no effect. This is normally the amount taken in a blood donor session.
Up to two litres (3.5 pints)	Hormones such as adrenaline are released, causing the pulse to increase and inducing sweating. Small blood vessels in non-vital areas, such as the skin, shut down to divert blood and oxygen to the vital organs. Signs of shock become evident.
Two litres (35 pints) or more(about one third of the usual volume in the average adult)	As blood or fluid loss approaches this level the radial pulse becomes difficult to find. The casualty will lose consciousness. Breathing may cease and the casualty may go into cardiac arrest.

Source: Kindleysides (2007)

mental health practitioner may be the first person at hand to help so they are in a key position to assess, implement BLS and hand over to emergency staff.

Clients who tell you they have overdosed

If clients report taking an overdose you should implement the emergency medical procedure. We cannot risk second guessing that the client is seeking attention by lying, as they may not be. If indeed they have then this will only be discovered following thorough examination and treatment. In this case it is always better to be safe than sorry.

Assessment of overdose

Ask the client:

- what type of substance(s) they have taken;
- how much of the substance(s) they have taken;
- when they took the substance(s);
- whether they have noticed any effects such as palpitations, sweating, dizziness;
- where the substance(s) were taken;
- whether anything else was taken.

Clients should be placed on one to one observations not only to ensure they do not take anything else, but to prevent any injury that might occur if they suddenly become unwell and faint. Baseline observations should be taken and documented at 15 minute intervals while awaiting transfer to the general hospital setting. Clients should not be allowed to eat or drink anything prior to a medical assessment.

Clients who have not told you and are found collapsed

Trying to discover why someone has collapsed is secondary to the immediate task of ensuring their immediate physical health and well-being. At times we can have an idea as in the previous example; other times we just have to provide emergency life support until the client is transferred to an acute care setting. Clients collapsed due to overdose will not be able to give us any information. So we must do the following:

- remember A, B, C;
- ensure basic first aid is provided;
- get medical/emergency help;
- arrange for immediate transfer;
- put into recovery position to prevent asphyxiation;
- check for evidence of anything that may have been ingested (blister packs or empty medicine bottles).

Following such incidents continuous observation and monitoring is important. This may include blood tests to check blood plasma levels of any medications that may have been taken, e.g. paracetamol. Clients will also need to know about the long term risks of the substances that they have overdosed on. For example liver damage is possible in adults who have taken 10g or more of paracetamol (MHRA 2009).

Intoxication

Clients will get intoxicated at times, either at home or in hospital. Our immediate concerns should be the client's physical safety rather than their reasons for drinking. Alcohol is a drug with powerful sedative effects that can depress the central nervous system (CNS). Psychotropic drugs also depress the CNS. Therefore a combination of both can be potentially life threatening as this can have adverse effects on cardiac and respiratory function. Most medication labels come with a warning advising abstinence during treatment. If a client returns to the ward intoxicated you should

- assess the severity of intoxication – take a breathalyser reading;
- elicit the type of substance used, e.g. alcohol or drugs (perform a urine/saliva drug test);
- inform the ward or duty doctor;
- remember A, B, C.

Intoxicated clients should be placed on bed rest. They should be positioned in the recovery position to prevent asphyxiation. They should also be supported, if possible, by bedsides to prevent accidental falls or placed on continuous observations. Baseline observations, focusing specifically on breathing and general state should be recorded routinely. This should be discussed with the doctor as it may be impractical to take blood pressure readings every fifteen minutes so this may be recorded at hourly or two hourly intervals. The doctor will also advise about medication, which may be withheld in the intervening period. If so ensure that this is clearly documented in the client case notes and medication chart.

For clients in the community it is not as easy to implement a plan of care such as this. Community practitioners need policy and organizational support on how to respond effectively to clients intoxicated at home. It would be unfair to place the onus on practitioners to develop plans as this may conflict with clinical governance standards of risk management. Organizational responses should be underpinned by the experience of practitioners. This would make for good policy and safe clinical decision making.

Box 9.5 Exercise   Which types of medical emergencies are covered in the unit medical emergency policy?

Can psychotropic medications cause medical emergencies?

Psychotropic medications can cause medical emergencies: although these events are considered rare, the possibility still exists. Psychotropic medications do not need to be taken in large quantities, as in overdose, to provoke a medical emergency. Chapter 8 explored adverse drug reactions that can occur on maintenance doses of medication. However, certain medications such as tricyclic antidepressants taken as an overdose can have fatal consequences. Sometimes when our clients are highly agitated they may require rapid tranquillization; this has been known to result in a medical emergency. This part of the chapter will explore medical emergencies linked to psychotropic medications, specifically

- lithium toxicity
- neuroleptic malignant syndrome
- serotonin syndrome
- rapid tranquillization

Lithium toxicity

Lithium has a very narrow therapeutic range making it easy for clients to suffer adverse effects. If these go undiagnosed they may lead to lithium toxicity which can be life threatening. Lithium toxicity is related to the concentration of lithium in blood plasma. However, side effects of lithium toxicity can occur even within therapeutic levels. The therapeutic range of lithium is 0.4–1mmol/l (BNF 2007).

Mild to moderate lithium intoxication can occur with levels above 1mmol/l. Signs of mild to moderate toxicity include

- gastro-intestinal symptoms – cramp, diarrhoea;
- neurological symptoms – hand tremor, disorientation, confusion, ataxia;
- blurred vision, thirst, drowsiness.

Moderate to severe intoxication can occur between 1.5–2mmol/l. Over 2mmol/l is a medical emergency and requires treatment indicated under emergency treatment of poisoning (BNF 2007). In addition to those above, signs of moderate to severe toxicity include

- renal impairment;
- muscle twitching, course hand tremor, nystagmus;
- severe vomiting and diarrhoea;
- seizures or coma;
- if untreated, certain death.

Treatment of lithium intoxication

In mild cases of intoxication, withdrawal of lithium and generous amounts of sodium salts and fluid will reverse toxicity and in severe cases treatment with haemodialysis might be required (BNF 2007). Activated charcoal is not used as it does not bind to lithium ions (Timmer and Sands 1999). Lithium intoxication may occur as an adverse drug reaction stemming from the maintenance use of lithium. However, severe poisoning occurs as a result of overdose. When overdose occurs the treatment of lithium poisoning is a priority. Timmer and Sands (1999) recommend:

- protect oral airway if consciousness is impaired;
- intravenous normal saline if volume depleted;
- whole bowel irrigation with polyethylene glycol (to prevent absorption);
- sodium polystyrene sulfonate (replaces lithium with sodium);
- haemodialysis
  - lithium level .6 mEq/L: any patient;
  - lithium level .4 mEq/L: any patient on chronic lithium therapy;
  - lithium level between 2.5 and 4 mEq/L: any patient with severe neurologic symptoms, renal insufficiency, or unstable hemodynamically or neurologically;
  - lithium level, 2.5 mEq/L: haemodialysis indicated only for patients with end-stage renal disease or patients whose lithium levels increase after admission or who fail to reach a lithium level below 1 mEq/L in 30 h.

In cases of overdose further advice should be sought from the National Poisons Information Service (http://www.npis.org).

Neuroleptic malignant syndrome

Neuroleptic malignant syndrome (NMS) is a life-threatening, neurological disorder caused by an adverse reaction to neuroleptic drugs. NMS has been described in association with all neuroleptic medications in current usage (Kohen and Bristow 1996). Rapid and large increases in dosage can trigger NMS.

NMS has been reported with non-neuroleptic drugs such as lithium, metoclopramide, carbamazepine, and antidepressants including dothiepin and amoxapine (Haddad 1994). Indeed Patel and Bristow (1987) report a case of NMS in a patient prescribed droperidol 5 mg and metoclopramide 10 mg IV as post-operative antiemetics. NMS is more prevalent in males than females and 90 per cent of cases begin within 10 days of the start of treatment with a neuroleptic drug, though not necessarily for the first time (Haddad 1994).

Risk factors for NMS

These include:

- previous history of NMS, known cerebral compromise;
- mental state: agitation, overactivity, catatonia;
- physical state: dehydration.

(Kohen and Bristow 1996)

Haddad (1994) suggests that the high fever may be due to the sustained rigidity and tremor that may produce considerable heat.

Management of NMS

NMS usually lasts for five to seven days but may be prolonged if depot antipsychotics have also been given (Keogh and Doyle 2008). Clinical management involves

- measurement of white cell count, electrolytes and urea, liver function and creatine phosphokinase (CPK);
- correcting dehydration and pyrexia;
- withdrawing neuroleptics, lithium and antidepressants;
- ECT and benzodiazepines not contraindicated;
- specific remedies (bromocryptine, dantrolene) are probably useful;
- referral to medical team.

(Kohen and Bristow 1996)

Differential diagnosis

Although NMS is rare we must be able to recognize it when it occurs. When considering a diagnosis of NMS you should consider differential diagnoses that can present with similar symptoms. These include catatonia, heat exhaustion, extrapyramidal symptoms with intermittent fever, partial NMS (neuro-toxicity falling below full blown NMS), thyrotoxic crisis and lupus (Kohen and Bristow 1996).

Serotonin syndrome

Serotonin is a neurotransmitter that effects sensory perception, temperature regulation, control of mood, appetite and the induction of sleep (Tortora and Derrickson 2006). Reduced levels of serotonin can lead to depression. This is because the neurones which release it take it back in so it only remains in the synapse for a short period. SSRI drugs are a frontline treatment of depressive illnesses as they prevent this 'reuptake'; hence the name – reuptake inhibitor. Therefore serotonin remains in the synapse longer, reducing feelings of depression.

Serotonin syndrome (SS) is a rare but life-threatening adverse reaction caused by an excess of serotonin. It can occur within the first 24 hours of taking the medication or when it has been increased (Keogh and Doyle 2008). The risk of SS increases when combinations of drugs, which act on the serotonin system, are given, for example, combining SSRI drugs with MAOIs (Murphy *et al.* 2004). Awareness of SS among prescribing doctors is poor. In a UK study, Mackay *et al.* (1999) found 85 per cent of general practitioners reported that they were unaware of the syndrome. This represents an area where community practitioners can offer education to primary care colleagues.

While SS is rare, practitioners should be familiar with the signs and symptoms in case they come across it. This will ensure prompt intervention. Knowing your client's medication regime will allow you to make a quick diagnosis as it is unlikely to be present in clients not taking serotonergic medications. Symptoms of SS affect the autonomic and motor systems and the way people behave. Three other major symptoms should be present before a diagnosis is made.

Murphy *et al.* (2004) categorize symptoms of serotonin syndrome as

- **autonomic** – tachycardia, hypertension, diaphoresis, fever progressing to hyperthermia;
- **motor** – shivering, myoclonus (involuntary twitching), tremor, hyper-reflexia, oculomotor abnormalities;
- **behavioural** – restlessness, agitation, delirium, coma.

Serotonin syndrome is a differential diagnosis of NMS as symptoms are very similar.

Management of serotonin syndrome

Isbister *et al.* (2007) suggest that serotonin toxicity can have three stages of severity – mild, moderate and severe. This helps to assess the level of intervention required. Initial management should begin with observation and screening and Mackay *et al.* (1999) suggest careful monitoring in the early clinical experience with new drugs. The management of SS will depend on its severity. Extreme cases may require intensive care with cardiac monitoring and mechanical ventilation (Murphy *et al.* 2004). In all cases all serotonergic medications should be discontinued. Keogh and Doyle (2008) suggest using cooling blankets, fans and so on for alleviating hyperthermia, drinking plenty of fluids and monitoring vital signs and urine output.

Rapid tranquillization

The aim of rapid tranquillization (RT) is to inhibit acute behavioural disturbances as quickly and safely as possible. This can be done by giving the client different types of medication in different modes. An agitated client will normally be offered oral medication in an attempt to calm them down. If this is refused and the situation cannot be effectively de-escalated, then intramuscular (IM) or intravenous (IV) medication may be given.

Taylor *et al.* (2005) state that the aims of RT are threefold:

- To reduce the suffering of the patient
- To reduce risk of harm to others by maintaining a safe environment
- To do no harm

In RT, medication is usually given as an IM preparation but sometimes, depending on the severity of the disturbance, IV preparations may be used. Types of medications that may be used either as IM or IV preparations include benzodiazepines, such as lorazepam or diazepam and antipsychotics, such as olanzapine, haloperidol and Clopixol Acuphase.

Antipsychotic drugs have cardiotoxic effects. When given as IV preparations this can lead to QT prolongation that can result in torsade de pointes and sudden death, for example, haloperidol can be given IV but it can cause cardiac arrest and death (Silva 1999). Lorazepam is used to calm agitated clients but this can cause severe respiratory depression. The BNF (2007) recommends that facilities for managing respiratory depression with mechanical ventilation must be at hand when IV medication is given.

NICE (2005) cautions staff to be aware of the potential results of RT:

- loss of consciousness instead of tranquillization;
- sedation with loss of alertness;
- loss of airway;
- cardiovascular and respiratory collapse;
- interaction with medicines already prescribed or illicit substances taken (can cause side effects such as akathisia, disinhibition);
- possible damage to patient–staff relationship;
- underlying coincidental physical disorders.

Box 9.6
Exercise   Describe the aftercare of someone who has had RT.

Effective safety measures must be in place to ensure the health and safety of clients and staff. For example, in restraint situations where medication is required there is a risk of needlestick injury to both clients and staff. It is important that the client is safely restrained to reduce the risk of a flailing limb leading to a needlestick injury. For practitioners working in forensic units or psychiatric intensive care wards training needs analysis in this area should be based on NICE (2005) guidance. Here all staff involved in the process of RT should receive ongoing competency training to a minimum of the Resuscitation Council UK's Immediate Life Support which covers airway, cardio-pulmonary resuscitation and the use of defibrillators (NICE 2005).

Conclusion

Medical emergencies are rare events that require immediate intervention to prevent deterioration and stabilize the client's health. This will stop when appropriate emergency services arrive and take over the emergency care of the client. Good clinical decision making and intervention in medical emergencies will be based on our knowledge of the client's physical health, whether they are currently being treated for a physical condition, their past medical history and current medication regime.

Summary of key points

- Practitioners should be aware of local policy and procedure for medical emergencies.
- Practitioners should be up to date with first aid and BLS training.
- Practitioners should be aware of adverse drug reactions that can result in medical emergency.

- Practitioners should reflect on the skills required to perform competently in an emergency situation.
- Practitioners should be up to date with using medical equipment such as pulse oximiter or defibrillator.

Quick quiz

1 List the factors that might induce a state of collapse.
2 What physical effects might be present in someone who has lost 2 litres of blood?
3 What are the early signs of hyperglycaemia?
4 List the type of equipment that might be required during a medical emergency.
5 List the symptoms of serotonin syndrome.

10 Practical steps in improving the physical health of people with severe mental illness

At the end of this chapter we will have:

- Explored the role of the nurse in improving physical health

- Examined the role of the practitioner in combating stigma and advocating for client rights

- Explored the public health role of the nurse in health education and promotion

- Examined NICE guidance that should support nursing practice

- Considered developing working relationships with other health care professionals

Introduction

Box 10.1 What is caseload profiling?
Exercise

'I'm a mental health nurse; physical health is not my job.' Such sentiments do exist, but gladly they are in a minority. Research shows that mental health nurses are highly motivated to attend physical health training (Nash 2005). In a descriptive study of 20 clients and 10 staff, Meddings and Perkins (2002) found that both groups had different perceptions about what getting better meant. Activities of daily living and access to help and support was rated more important by practitioners whereas clients rated improved material and physical well-being as more important. Although a small study, it does show that our clients are interested in their physical health.

Facilitating physical health and well-being is a complex task that will cross different boundaries, for example, health and education providers, mental health and primary care services, even the inter-professional team. Yet it is not unrealistic to expect that our clients can have good standards of physical health care that can increase their quality of life. Clients' interest in their physical health and practitioners' motivation for training are powerful drivers for change. However, these need to be harnessed in order to influence organizational behaviour and policy. Much of the work required has already been done with the many national service frameworks and NICE guidelines (see Table 10.1). These require integration into the organization and delivery of our clients' care to improve their health and well-being.

Physical health and well-being is a neglected area of mental health care. Our main goals for physical health and well-being are not complex. They should be

- keeping our clients healthy;
- preventing our clients from becoming ill;
- when our clients become ill, minimizing the impact of this and strive to make them better as quickly as possible.

These goals are reasonable enough to be adopted as general principles, or philosophies of physical health care. Indeed there is a policy initiative stemming from the UK Chief Nursing Officer's review of mental health nursing (DH 2006). This recommends that we focus on improving the physical well-being of people with severe mental health problems. As we have seen in this book very simple, measurable targets can be set that can ensure an evidence base for practice. This will provide measures for the effectiveness of our individual or organizational interventions. Targets should include:

- Reducing obesity
- Reducing smoking
- Increasing physical activity
- Promoting positive health and well-being through immunizations and screening
- Decreasing alcohol consumption
- Monitoring adverse drug reactions

Table 10.1 Key National Service Framework (NSF) aims and standards for health improvement and prevention

CHD
Standard one
The NHS and partner agencies should develop, implement and monitor policies that reduce the prevalence of coronary risk factors in the population, and reduce inequalities in risks of developing heart disease.
Standard two
The NHS and partner agencies should contribute to a reduction in the population in the prevalence of smoking in the local population.
Mental Health
Standard one
Health and social services should:
• promote mental health for all, working with individuals and communities
• combat discrimination against individuals and groups with mental health problems and promote social inclusion.
The Cancer Plan
The Cancer Plan sets out aims to:
• reduce the risk of cancer through reducing smoking and promoting a healthier diet
• raise public awareness with better, more accessible information.
Diabetes
Standard one
The NHS will develop, implement and monitor strategies to reduce the risk of developing type 2 diabetes in the population as a whole and to reduce the inequalities in the risk of developing type 2 diabetes.
Older People
As well as older people having access to all of the above, the NSF sets out health promotion activities which are of specific benefit to older people:
• increasing physical activity
• improved diet and nutrition
• immunisation and management programmes for influenza
• requirements for preventing falls and strokes.

Source: Department of Health (2002a), reproduced with permission

By focusing on these priorities we can reduce the burden of ill health on individuals, families and health services. These targets will impact on rates of heart disease, respiratory disease and diabetes, which are very prevalent in our client group. Tackling inequalities in health may be more difficult to achieve but not impossible. Mental health services should be liaising strategically with primary care services in respect to commissioning physical care services. Practitioners should advocate on behalf of clients to get access to primary care services: this will help reduce inequalities in care.

We will address what can be done in relation to physical health and well-being in three distinct ways:

- what individual practitioners can do
- what mental health services can do
- what education and training providers can do

Box 10.2 Exercise	How is the NSF for diabetes or the NICE guidelines for diabetes implemented in the care of your clients?

What can individual practitioners do?

The review of mental health nursing in the UK (DH 2006) recommends that nurses have the skills to improve clients' physical well-being (see Table 10.2). Practitioners and organizations have a mutual dependence in meeting these needs. In this difficult economic period training budgets are usually the first to get raided to pay for services. However, this is short-sighted management. Investment in skills and the workforce will bring better long term sustainable

Table 10.2 Recommendation 7 from the Chief Nursing Officer's review of mental health nursing

Recommendation 7: MHNs will have the skills and opportunities to improve the physical well-being of people with mental health problems.

Making change happen	Key contributors
1 MHNs to have the appropriate competencies to support physical well-being through: • Assessment of current capabilities in teams and developing team-based training based on local need; and/or • Developing individual development programmes based on individual appraisal using the Knowledge and Skills framework.	**Service providers** with MHNs, line managers, education leads and supervisors.
2 MHNs to be able to: • Refer on to medical or other primary care staff in response to evidence of unmet physical health need, arranging support as required to ensure services are then actually received; or • Arrange for further investigations themselves.	**All MHNs** with clinical supervisors, line managers, clinical governance departments, other professionals and healthcare organizations.
3 MHNs to identify the need for and provide, or refer for, health promotion information and activities required to support physical well-being.	

Source: Department of Health (2006), reproduced with permission

gains. Practitioners can still work at the micro client–practitioner level, even though there is instability in the macro economic level.

Role of mental health nurse

The role of the mental health nurse may change depending on the specific context of practice. For example, in inpatient settings there will be a better opportunity for increased health surveillance than community settings by virtue of clients being in hospital. However, the broad principles of roles are similar (see Figure 10.1).

Screening and identifying physical illness

Acute inpatient nurses spend a lot of time with clients and are in a good position to screen and identify physical health needs and initiate health promotion activities, e.g. smoking cessation. They are also in a good position to work jointly with dieticians in planning healthy eating programmes. Similarly, community mental health nurses can facilitate physical screening in line with NICE guidelines for schizophrenia and bipolar disorder.

Screening is part of the process of caseload profiling. Here the prevalence of health problems is mapped. Practitioners need to have basic skills in screening for physical illness. These skills stem from knowledge of risk factors covered in this book and the ability to identify these in clients. Practitioners already working with those who have a diagnosed physical condition may feel it necessary to supplant general skills with more specialist ones. Clinical audit will be an important factor in putting this information to use in commissioning health care, developing services and identifying staff training needs.

Profiling the health of your caseload

Caseload profiling is a practical step that can be taken in beginning the process of facilitating physical health and well-being. To begin you will need to develop a caseload auditing tool (see the example in Table 10.3; also refer to Chapter 2). Profiling is a form of health needs assessment. Hooper and Longworth (2002: 9) define health needs assessment (HNA) as 'a systematic and explicit process which reviews the health issues affecting a population. The process aims to improve health, and reduce health inequalities, by identifying local priorities

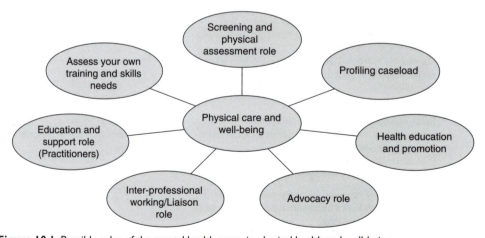

Figure 10.1 Possible roles of the mental health nurse in physical health and well-being

Table 10.3 Example of a caseload profile audit tool

Factor	Variable	Rationale
Demographics	Gender, ethnicity, age, employment status, marital status	Demographic characteristics can help to identify specific at risk groups and explore exposure to risk factors or physical conditions, e.g. smoking rates in men or diabetes risk in clients from ethnic minorities
Physical illness	Current diagnosis Signs and symptoms	To ensure effective clinical management Screening for signs and symptoms of undiagnosed physical illness, e.g. monitoring blood cholesterol levels
Psychiatric diagnosis	Current diagnosis	Some diagnoses may increase risk of physical illness, e.g. schizophrenia can increase risk of diabetes
Exposure to risk factors	Presence of current risk factors such as smoking, alcohol/drug use, obesity, sedentary lifestyle	To map the need for treatments, e.g. how many clients want smoking cessation, or which client(s) may require statins or oral hypoglycaemic agents
Current medications	Risk of metabolic disorders, risk of cardiac disorders, risk of toxicity	Medication regimes require effective monitoring, e.g. monitoring lithium levels in clients with bi-polar disorder
Substance use	Current alcohol use Current drug use	To identify specific problems related to this

for change and then planning the actions needed to make these changes happen.' HNA can be facilitated at an individual practitioner or ward level. Ideally this should be a strategic initiative across all parts of the organization so that more accurate needs profiles can be developed.

Following profiling unmet needs can be examined. For example, the rate of clients with elevated blood cholesterol levels who are not currently prescribed statins or the availability of smoking cessation aids and nicotine replacement therapy for clients who want to quit smoking. However, unmet needs are not just medical, they may also be social, e.g. ensuring clients have the appropriate state benefits with which they may be able to include more healthy foods in their diet; or organizational, e.g. having occupational therapy and dietician input to support dietary changes.

Health education and promotion

We have a key role to play in preventing physical ill health as we may be the only person the client engages with. Our clients are among the most vulnerable groups in society and face enormous social exclusion. For example, we know from research that people with SMI face problems in primary care that range from their physical health not being wholly assessed (Kendrick 1996) or exclusion from GP lists (Buntwal et al. 1999). However, even when in contact with health services their physical needs may be neglected by diagnostic overshadowing or practitioners not having appropriate physical care skills or training (Nash 2005).

When embarking on health promotion activities practitioners need to have an idea of models of health promotion in order to understand the challenges that clients face. This knowledge will help with tailoring individual plans for clients. A popular health promotion model is Prochaska and DiClemente's (1983) stages of change model outlined below:

- Pre-contemplation – clients do not see the need for change, or some don't want to change or some are unaware that they need to change.
- Contemplation – clients are aware of problems but are ambivalent about addressing them.
- Preparation – clients are ready to change or have tried to change, i.e. 'testing the water'.
- Action – clients have taken action, e.g. they have gone to a smoking cessation group.
- Maintenance – clients need practitioners to support them so that change can be fostered and positive lifestyle changes built upon.
- Relapse is also a stage to consider. Lifestyle change is difficult and clients may relapse a few times before they finally quit smoking. It is important that we give support to clients in this stage so that we can empower them to regain action.

Opportunistic health promotion

Opportunistic health promotion is a practical way to begin the process of health promotion. We are all in contact with clients and carers at some stage of our work. Therefore we should take the opportunity to use this client contact to raise consciousness about positive physical health. This can be employed in inpatient areas where clients are easy to reach or in the community, out-patient or other clinics.

Box 10.3 Exercise	Examine the contents of your ward notice board or client information packs. Is there an opportunity of including health promotion material here?

A crude audit of our areas will probably find more information about various take-away menus than healthy eating materials. The vending machines in or around our areas will have a disproportionate amount of high calorie snack bars and fizzy drinks than healthy alternatives. We need to redress this imbalance. In the UK each primary care trust has a health promotion unit that has lots of useful resources that can be used to raise consciousness. These may have a minimal cost or may even be free of charge. For example, posters beside elevators encouraging people to use the stairs is one way of promoting gentle exercise and posters reminding clients to reduce salt intake or eat more fruit and vegetables can promote healthy eating.

Advocating for clients' rights

Advocacy is important for securing the rights of access to proper physical health care for clients in both hospital and primary care settings. Roberts *et al.* (2007) conducted a case note review to determine whether patients with a diagnosis of schizophrenia receive the same levels of physical health care from primary care practitioners as patients without schizophrenia. They found that clients with schizophrenia were less likely to have smoking status noted and less likely to have either blood pressure or cholesterol recorded. They conclude that clients with a diagnosis of schizophrenia are less likely to receive some important general health checks than patients without schizophrenia, even though they have increased health risks. While these results appear dispiriting, they do provide an opportunity for us to either advocate more strongly on behalf of our clients; empower them to be more autonomous when visiting their GP; or increase our liaison and support of primary care colleagues.

Advocating for clients' rights will be a central aim of facilitating physical health and well-being. While this will happen across all types of services it will be of particular significance for practitioners working in community settings or with vulnerable client groups.

Inter-professional working/liaison role

Most of our clients will have complex health needs. This complexity requires effective management to ensure best practice and efficient use of resources. Good communication will be a key part of this as facilitating physical care has to be achieved in a holistic way. Inter-professional working is required to ensure that the client gets the best assessment and care plan. Meeting needs should be a shared responsibility between primary care and mental health. Financial rewards are not the only rewards; there is also access to training and the scope to develop innovative practice.

Nurse-led chronic disease management is part of the everyday workload for many practice nurses and nurse practitioners (Louch 2005). Therefore ensuring our clients are able to access these clinics when they need to will require effective inter-professional working and liaison. Partnership working with primary care colleagues will be a vital component of the physical health agenda. This partnership working is already recognized in shared care arrangements for addressing the care of people with severe mental illness. Most community mental health nurses will have good working links with GP practices in their locality. Therefore this will be a natural extension of these links. What is now required is reciprocity in the shared physical care of people with severe mental illness.

All mental health practitioners have a role in developing the physical care agenda. Mental health nurses are already skilled at inter-professional team-working so the challenge may not be so great. Nevertheless, there will probably be tensions in a range of areas, e.g. between the use of the medical model to drive change rather than a social model; tension between managers and practitioners regarding rewards or resources; or between primary care and mental health services around whose responsibility it is to fund this developing agenda.

Assessing your learning needs in physical health and well-being

Nursing is a profession which requires its members to engage in continuous professional development in order to extend practice and offer high quality care to our clients. To achieve this effectively we must ensure that we are up to date with our knowledge and skills. This will ensure competence to practise safely. While predominantly an individual responsibility our employers also share in this by providing us access to appropriate education and training.

Research shows that mental health nurses may be using and depending on skills gained during their student nurse training – skills that may consequently not be up to date (Nash 2005). In an unpublished research project exploring qualified mental health nurses' knowledge of basic concepts in physical health, (Nash 2008) found general unawareness of fundamental aspects of physical health. For example, only 5 of the sample of 88 knew the therapeutic level of lithium. However, such issues are not confined to nursing. Phelan *et al.* (2001) state many mental health practitioners have little training in physical care and some experienced psychiatrists would probably admit to not having used a stethoscope or done a physical exam for a number of years. The lack of evidence relating to the physical care training needs of mental health professionals is surprising and it is important that this is borne in mind when appraisal or training needs are being considered for continuing professional development.

Training Needs Analysis

Pedder (1998) defines Training Needs Analysis (TNA) as being part of a strategic training plan where 'training or learning objectives are established, knowledge is mapped, gaps are identified and appropriate action is taken to meet needs'. TNA is one way in which organizations can measure the training and skills needs of practitioners to meet the physical health and well-being agenda. This would normally be done through a training audit. However, practitioners can undertake their own TNA as a way of identifying their own training needs. It is important that the TNA is realistic as the primary aim is to increase knowledge and skills to help meet the physical health and well-being needs of clients and increase the quality of their care rather than being a means to an end for staff development. As such the TNA will be strategic as it will aim to meet both the needs of clients for high quality care and practitioners in developing their scope for practice.

The TNA should be linked to the physical health and well-being needs of your client group. Therefore in analysing your training needs you may also be recognizing the physical health and well-being needs of your clients. How you prioritize importance will depend on your client group and any commitments to physical health that your organization has made. Prioritizing your training needs will relate either to the prevalence of physical conditions in your client group, e.g. a high prevalence of diabetes might indicate an area for training or to the prevalence of risk factors, e.g. a high prevalence of smoking might indicate a training need in smoking cessation.

Training recommendations may have a very specific context. For example, for practitioners who have clients taking lithium, an important training need would be the recognition of lithium toxicity and how to manage this. For practitioners working in forensic, or other types of secure services, a TNA may look to develop skills for physical health and well-being during and following restraint or rapid tranquillization.

Box 10.4 Case example

Sheila is a staff nurse working in a rehabilitation setting. She has been qualified for ten years and has extensive experience in Cognitive Behavioural Therapy for psychosis. There is a new policy in her unit which focuses on the physical health and well-being needs of clients. Sheila has grown concerned at her lack of skills in physical health care. She has noticed some of her client group are overweight, smoke excessively, take little exercise and all are on atypical antipsychotic medication; factors the policy highlights as risks to physical health. She needs to begin writing care plans that aim to tackle these risks but is not confident in her physical care planning skills.

This scenario is not that uncommon in either inpatient or community practice. First, Sheila has kept up to date with her mental health nursing skills but has not undertaken any training in physical health and well-being. This is not unusual as being an expert practitioner in mental health is a common goal for us all. Facilitating physical health and well-being is a relatively new area of training need where specific courses have only recently been available. Sheila recognizes that she needs to improve her physical care skills as there is a new unit policy. Sheila also notices certain risk factors for physical illness in her client group. Combining all of these factors she can reflect on how best she can express her perceived learning and skills needs and discuss these with her clinical supervisor, or manager as part of the individual performance review.

Box 10.5 Case example continued

Sheila meets with her manager for a performance review. She has identified training needs required to implement the local policy and provide good client care. She discusses these with her manager who is supportive of her identified training needs in the following areas

- Physical health assessment
- Screening for physical illness to include clinical observation skills
- Skills for health education and health promotion
- Managing the physical side effects of psychotropic medication

Your own TNA will be influenced by

- rates of current physical morbidity;
- prevalence of risk factors for physical illness;
- the clinical skills you need to facilitate physical health and well-being.

Box 10.6   Conduct your own brief TNA related to the physical health and well-being needs of
Exercise   your clients.

Education and support

Primary care practitioners generally lack awareness of mental health problems. This not only relates to specific conditions but also to the problems caused by stigma, labelling and stereotyping. A challenge for community nurses is educating primary care workers about how these can increase risks to our client's physical health. The lifestyle risks will be easy to illustrate as these will be a common feature of their everyday work. However, they may not have had education that addresses stigma as a risk that can lead to social exclusion and how this impacts on the physical health of clients. Challenging negative attitudes and stigma will be important in reducing health inequalities and increasing access to primary care services.

Clinical supervision is another area where mental health nurses can offer support to primary care colleagues. Increasing support to non-mental health workers can increase their confidence and ability to work with our clients. Just providing some training and leaving it at that may not engender ownership of any change that is required. However, providing support through clinical supervision can increase confidence, inter-professional working, promote networking and explore avenues for further practice developments.

What can mental health services do?

Mental health managers must ensure that resources are available to meet and sustain the policy agenda for facilitating physical health and well-being. This will entail strategic discussions between mental health services and primary care providers to determine:

- whose responsibility is it to meet the physical health care needs of clients;
- what are the roles of respective staff in facilitating physical health and well-being;
- how clients can get timely access to primary care services;
- what can be done to support primary care staff in working with clients.

Most mental health facilities should also have some form of physical health and well-being strategy. This strategy will have measurable targets that can be audited, e.g. all clients will have a physical assessment within 42 hours of admission.

Mental health services also need to develop commissioning frameworks in order to utilize scarce resources effectively. Some might believe that our role in commissioning will be negligible. However, the commissioning process will be informed by profiling our caseloads and prioritizing health needs assessment (see Figure 10.2). Even if the decision is that there are no resources to meet the identified needs, we should not allow these decisions to be made easily. Generating evidence will put the issues into the policy arena and once there, they will not go away. At some stage the resources will have to come.

Annual health checks

Mental health services, in conjunction with primary care, should instigate a programme of annual health checks for clients. While resource implications may make this target difficult to achieve, it should not be impossible with effective holistic care. This is where we have to target our clients effectively in order to produce health gains. For example we could begin by considering annual health checks on clients with bipolar disorder as recommended by NICE (2006a).

People with severe mental illness should be routinely and systematically health screened as part of a holistic care programme. Some of this screening may be gender specific, e.g. cervical smear screening for women, and should be facilitated with close joint working and liaison with primary care services. This systematic screening should focus on the recognized 'big killers' of CHD, cancers and obesity, with respiratory screening also included for asthma and other respiratory disorders.

Rethink Policy Statement 36 (Took 2001) advocates at least annual physical health checks. Physical health should not be seen in isolation at client reviews and the integration of physical care, as part of the UK Care Programme Approach process or other case review, would make the process truly holistic. Of course there are resource implications in relation to training mental health professionals in physical assessment and management skills. However, such issues have to be considered in respect of the benefits of increased physical health of our clients, their satisfaction with our services and our closer working with primary health care colleagues.

One aspect of the annual health check will be general health education and health promotion advice. This will be aimed at promoting a healthy lifestyle and include

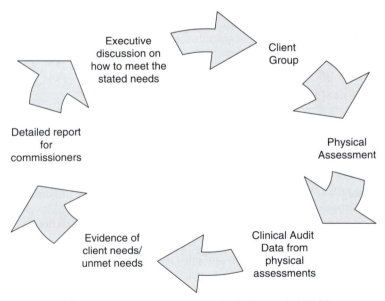

Figure 10.2 How mental health nurses can influence commissioning physical health care

- smoking cessation
- diet and nutrition
- sexual health
- oral hygiene
- exercise
- alcohol and/or drug use

The annual health check should also include

- immunization – flu and/or pneumococcal, TB
- allergies
- screening for cervical or prostate cancer
- self screening of testes or breasts for lumps

There is no real consensus on what an annual health check should consist of as there is always the question of resources in relation to two factors:

- having the necessary equipment to carry out an assessment;
- whose responsibility it is to meet identified health needs.

Table 10.4 gives an example of an annual health check.

Table 10.4 Example of an annual health check

Area	Clinical observation
General observations	Temperature, blood pressure, pulse, respirations
Cardiac assessment	ECG
Respiratory assessment	Peak flow for asthma sufferers
Endocrine assessment	Urinalysis Blood glucose levels Thyroid function test
Weight	BMI Waist circumference Waist hip ratio
Lifestyle factors	Smoking Alcohol/drug use Exercise
Blood screening	Full blood count Blood glucose Blood cholesterol Regular monitoring of medication levels Hepatitis status
Public health	Sexual health advice Immunizations
Adverse drug reactions	Review of metabolic and coronary adverse drug reactions Review of other adverse drug reactions Use NICE guidance and BNF guidelines to develop medication review criteria
Other aresa	Oral health Hearing and sight tests Skin integrity

Box 10.7 Exercise	Think of your client group and the physical illnesses they have. What can you do to prevent these conditions from getting worse? How can you prevent others from developing similar conditions?

Logistics in prioritizing annual health checks will need to be local as the same arrangements may be difficult to implement in inner city and rural areas. It would be possible for the CPA to be used to facilitate the annual health check. For example, it can be performed prior to discharge and then yearly for clients being discharged from hospital. For community clients it may be performed during various reviews. Table 10.5 illustrates the decisions that may be required about when, where, how and by whom an annual health check is undertaken.

The role of education providers

The stereotypical view of academics in ivory towers rings true when education provision does not keep a pace with shifts in clinical practice. Physical health and well-being is one area where

Table 10.5 Factors to consider when implementing an annual health check

Goal	All clients, inpatient and community, require an annual physical health check

Priority	Clients already diagnosed with physical conditions
	Clients with severe mental illness
	Clients with severe mental illness treated with poly-pharmacy:
	    Clients with severe mental illness taking two or more antipsychotic drugs
	    Clients taking lithium and an antipsychotic drug
	    Clients taking antipsychotics and benzodiazepines
	    Clients taking antipsychotic and antidepressant medication
	    Clients being treated over the BNF recommended daily levels of drugs
	Clients with substance misuse problems:
	    Clients injecting substances
	    Clients taking multiple substances
	    Clients on methadone maintenance programmes
	Clients with multiple physical health risk factors:
	    Policy related targets e.g. priority is given to screening for the big killers like heart disease and cancer
	Clients from some minority ethnic backgrounds
	Clients with a family history of medical illness

Action	Physical health check on admission may double as an annual health check Physical health check on discharge may double as an annual health check Physical health check performed as part of the Care Programme Approach may double as the annual physical health check
Resources	Equipment Training Clinical standards
Responsibility	Responsible medical officer GP Care manager Key worker Primary nurse

education providers seem to have been caught napping. However, this is changing rapidly and a range of courses and study days are now available in universities, e.g. Middlesex University in London has developed physical care skills courses for mental health nurses.

While education providers need to be able to respond quickly to changes in clinical practice this should not be at the expense of quality. Education providers must not produce ad hoc courses that are not sustainable. The rush to provide anything can result in a diffusion of courses that quickly close because of low student numbers or poor quality. Being proactive and leading policy is better than being reactive and playing catch-up with it. The ability to respond quickly will stem from service providers and education providers having a close working relationship. Here education providers have a lot to learn from the different models and practices of working across boundaries that health care providers use daily. Closer joint working should involve educational in-reach which will see the education provider jointly involved in TNA so that identified local needs can be translated in to high quality courses that are relevant to learners' needs.

Joint research and audit can also be undertaken which will strengthen the strategic links between education providers and service providers which in turn can underpin commitments to lifelong learning. Here both parties with different types of resources can explore innovation in educational delivery. For example, universities have virtual learning environments such as WebCT and there must be some way that service providers can get access to the resources held there.

Education providers already have a portfolio of physical care courses for adult colleagues. Developing mental health specific versions of each would be unnecessary duplication of work. However, some inter-school cooperation could see variations of courses for mental health nurses or adult nursing academics involved in mental health teaching. For example, a respiratory care lecturer should be involved in respiratory assessment and airway management in the use of physical restraint. Undoubtedly there are many such examples.

The effectiveness of such interventions should be the subject of joint research. For example, does the provision of physical health education have an effect on the physical health and well-being of service users? Education providers should realize that the end recipients of their training courses are not the students in the classroom but the clients in their living room.

Box 10.8 **Exercise**	Take a few moments to reflect on your clinical practice. Which skills do you feel you need in order to provide physical care to your client group?

Challenges to meeting the physical health care agenda

Stigma is probably the biggest barrier to facilitating physical health and well-being in clients. Robson and Gray (2007: 458) suggest that mental health nurses are in a strategic position to have a positive impact on the mental and physical well-being of people with severe mental illness. Mental health nurses have a big role in combating stigma and challenging the negative attitudes and stereotypes that dog our client group. Stigma leads to social exclusion, which can result in clients not accessing services. Practitioners working in the community will have a role in advocating and educating primary care colleagues. We also all have a responsibility to challenge negative stereotypes that our colleagues might have regarding their own clients' physical health or ability to change lifestyle factors.

There are many complex reasons why practitioners may resist undertaking a physical care role. For example, if a practitioner has low levels of confidence in assessing physical health they may be disinclined to do it. The more they disengage from this area of work the higher the risk that they defer this to others and the opportunity for learning, or relearning, and extending practice is lost. For many of us it may have been a long time since we either had any training, or practice, in physical health care. This might make us a little reluctant to undertake this again, as the 'you can't teach an old dog new tricks' idea may inhibit us once more. For some practitioners there may be a partisan argument that as mental health specialists we should not undertake a physical health role as it is outside our scope of practice.

Sometimes practitioners are not rewarded for extending their roles or undertaking training and in light of this they may be dissuaded from engaging with the physical health agenda. Whatever the argument we can be sure that there will be losers on both sides. Clients may not get the holistic care that they need and mental health nurses limit their scope of practice, breadth of knowledge and development of new skills. The purpose here is not to argue for a generic medical/psychiatric workforce, but for us to develop competent skills in the recognition of symptoms of physical illness, the assessment of physical health and the referral onto more specialist services when something significant is uncovered.

Conclusion

We have a professional and ethical responsibility to remain up to date with our knowledge and skills. However, this is a responsibility that should be shared between practitioners and their organization. Organizations have the responsibility to provide training to practitioners but practitioners have a duty to utilize this for the benefit of clients. Extending our role in relation to facilitating physical health and well-being will be dependent on

- identifying appropriate training needs;
- linking these training needs to our client group;
- having resources and support to underpin new roles; and
- development of specialist education and training.

If this is commenced in a strategic way it should lead to the delivery of high standards of physical health care for our clients.

Summary of key points

- Mental health nurses have a key role in implementing and sustaining the physical health care agenda.
- Practitioners should identify their learning needs in conjunction with their clients' physical health and well-being needs.
- Organizations should support staff for long term development rather than short term gain.
- Education providers and service providers need to work closely to develop a sustainable physical health training agenda.

Quick quiz

1 Think about your client group and the work you do. How might your own levels of knowledge and skills act as a barrier to effective care?

2 How do you think clients and carers can be actively involved in the process of facilitating physical health and well-being?

3 How would you deal with stigmatizing attitudes towards clients?

4 Can you identify someone who could offer you clinical supervision and support around the area of facilitating physical health and well-being?

5 List examples of good practice in your clinical area.

References

Aboderin, I., Kalache, A., Ben-Shlomo, Y., *et al.* (2002) *Life Course Perspectives on Coronary Heart Disease, Stroke and Diabetes: Key Issues and Implications for Policy and Research*. Geneva: WHO.

Access Economics (2007) *Executive Summary Smoking and Mental Illness: Cost*. A report by Access Economic for SANE. http://www.health.wa.gov.au/smokefree/docs/SANE_Access_Economics_exec_summary.pdf, accessed 5 December, 2008.

Acheson, D. (1998) *Independent Inquiry into Inequalities in Health Report*. London: The Stationery Office.

Adams, J., Wilson, D.H, Taylor, A.W., *et al.* (2004) Psychological factors and asthma quality of life: a population based study, *Thorax*, 59: 930–5.

Alberti K.G.M.M., Zimmet, P. and Shaw, J. (2007) Review article International Diabetes Federation: a consensus on Type 2 diabetes prevention, *Diabetic Medicine*, 24: 451–63.

Alcohol Concern (2003) *Factsheet 6: Wernicke-Korsakoff Syndrome*. London: Alcohol Concern.

Allebeck, P. (1989) Schizophrenia: a life shortening disease, *Schizophrenia Bulletin*, 15: 81–9.

Allibone, L. and Nation, N. (2006) A guide to regulation of blood gases: part two, *Nursing Times*, 102(46) 48–50.

Amador, X. (2001) Anosognosia keeps patients from realizing they're ill, *Psychiatric News*, 36(17) 12.

American Diabetes Association, American Psychiatric Association, American Association of Clinical Endocrinologists, North American Association for the Study of Obesity (2004) Consensus development conference on antipsychotic drugs and obesity and diabetes, *Diabetes Care*, 27(2): 596–601.

American Psychiatric Association (1994) *Diagnostic and Statistical Manual of Mental Disorders (DSM-IV)*, 4th edn. Washington, DC: APA.

Anderson, K. and Anderson, L. (1995) *Mosby's Pocket Dictionary of Nursing, Medicine and Professions Allied to Medicine UK Edition*. London: Mosby.

Appleby, L., Thomas, S., Ferrier, N., *et al.* (2000) Sudden unexplained death in psychiatric in-patients, *The British Journal of Psychiatry*, 176: 405–6.

Asthma UK (2004) *Factfile Nebulisers and Asthma*, August 2004. http://www.asthma.org.uk/all_about_asthma/medicines_treatments/nebulisers.html, accessed 22 July 2009.

Australian Institute of Health and Welfare Australia's Health (2006) 2006AIHW Cat no. AUS73. Canberra: AIHW.

BAPEN (2008) *Malnutrition Universal Screening Tool* (MUST), http://www.bapen.org.uk/pdfs/must/must_full.pdf, accessed 22 July 2009.

Barnes, T., Paton, C., Cavanagh, M.R., Hancock, E. and Taylor, D. (on behalf of the UK Prescribing Observatory for Mental Health) (2007) A UK audit of screening for the metabolic side effects of antipsychotics in community patients, *Schizophrenia Bulletin*, 33(6) 1397–403.

Bennett, C. (2003a) Recording peak expiratory flow rate (PEFR), in B. Workman and C. Bennett, *Key Nursing Skills*. London: Whurr.

Bennett, C. (2003b) Respiratory care, in B. Workman and C. Bennett, *Key Nursing Skills*. London: Whurr.

Bennett, J., Done, J., Harrison-Read, P. *et al.* (1995) Development of a rating scale: check list to assess the side-effects of antipsychotics by Community Psychiatric Nurses, in C. Brooker and E. White (eds) *Community Psychiatric Nursing: A Research* Perspective (Vol. 3) London: Chapman and Hall.

Blaxter, M. (1990) *Health and Lifestyles*. London: Routledge.

BNF (British National Formulary) (2007) *No. 53*. British Medical Association and the Royal Pharmaceutical Society of Great Britain March 2007.

Booker, R. (2005) Chronic obstructive pulmonary disease: non pharmacological approaches, *British Journal of Nursing*, 14(1) 14–18.

Booker, R. (2007) Peak expiratory flow measurement, *Nursing* Standard, 21(39) 42–3.

Bradshaw, J. (1972) A taxonomy of social need, *New Society*, 30: 640–3, March.

Brashers, V.L. and Huether, S.E. (2004) Structure and function of the pulmonary system, in S.E. Huether and K.L. McCance (eds) (2004) *Understanding Pathophysiology*, 3rd edn. Edinburgh: Mosby.

British Heart Foundation (2004) *The Heart: Technical Terms Explained*, Heart Information Series Number 18. London: British Heart Foundation.

British Heart Foundation (2005a) *Blood Pressure*, Heart Information Series Number 4. London: British Heart Foundation.

British Heart Foundation (2005b) *Fact File Ventricular Arrhythmias*. London: British Heart Foundation.

British Heart Foundation (2006) *Angina Heart Information*. Series Number 6. London: British Heart Foundation.

British Heart Foundation (2007a) *Fact File No.5: Ethnic Differences in Cardiovascular Risk*. London: British Heart Foundation.

British Heart Foundation (2007b) *Atrial Fibrillation*. London: British Heart Foundation.

British Heart Foundation (2007c) *Medicines for the Heart*. Health Information Series No. 17. London: British Heart Foundation.

British Heart Foundation (2008a) *Cardioversion*. London: British Heart Foundation.

British Heart Foundation (2008b) *Heart Block*. London: British Heart Foundation.

British Hypotension Society (2006) *Blood Pressure Management*, Fact file 01/2006.

British Nutrition Foundation (2004) *The Metabolic Syndrome*, http://www.nutrition.org.uk/home.asp?siteId=43andsectionId=729andsubSectionId=327andparentSection=301andwhich=3, accessed 22 July 2009.

British Thoracic Society (2006) *The Burden of Lung Disease*, a Statistics Report from the British Thoracic Society, 2nd edn. London: BMJ.

British Thoracic Society (2008) Pharmacological management, in *British Guideline on the Management of Asthma: A National Clinical Guideline*. *Thorax* 63, Supplement IV iv1–iv1, 21 May.

Brown, M.C., Brown, J.D., Bayer, M.M. (1987) Changing nursing practice through continuing education in physical assessment: perceived barriers to implementation, *Journal of Continuing Education in Nursing*, 18(4) 11–15.

Brown, S., Birtwistle, J., Roe, L. *et al.* (1999) The unhealthy lifestyle of people with schizophrenia, *Psychological Medicine*, 29: 697–701.

Buchfa, V.L. and Fries, C.M. (2004) Respiratory care, in E.J. Mills (ed.) *Nursing Procedures*. Philadelphia: Lippincott Williams and Wilkins.

Buffington, S. and Turner, M. (2004) Part 3. Specimen collection and testing: urine specimens, in E.J. Mills (ed.) *Nursing Procedures*, 4th edn. Lippincott Williams and Wilkins.

Buntwal, N., Hare, J. and King, M. (1999) The struck-off mystery, *Journal of the Royal Society of Medicine*, 92(9) 443–5.

Burns, T. and Cohen, A. (1998) Item of Service payments for general practitioner care of severely mentally ill patients: does the money matter? *British Journal of General Practice*, 48: 1415–16.

Bushe, C. and Holt, R. (2004) Prevalence of diabetes and impaired glucose tolerance in patients with schizophrenia, *British Journal of Psychiatry*, 184: s67–s71.

Callaghan, P. (2004) Exercise: a neglected intervention in mental health care? *Journal of Psychiatric and Mental Health Nursing*, 11: 476–83.

Cancer Research UK (2006) Poisonous smoke, available at http://info.cancerresearchuk.org/healthyliving/smokeispoison/poisonoussmoke/?a=5441, accessed 20 November 2008.

Canoy, D., Matthijs Boekholdt, S., Wareham, N., *et al.* (2007) Epidemiology: body fat distribution and risk of coronary heart disease in men and women in the European prospective investigation into cancer and nutrition in Norfolk cohort: a population-based prospective study, *Circulation*, 116: 2933–43.

Cassidy, F., Ahearn, E. and Carroll, B.J. (1999) Elevated frequency of Diabetes Mellitus in hospitalized manic-depressive patients, *American Journal of Psychiatry*, 156: 1417–20.

Ch 10M (2008) Mental health student nurses' attitudes towards and experiences of the use of cigarettes to motivate patient behaviour. Unpublished research paper.

Chief Medical Officer (2004) *Tobacco and Borders: Death Made Cheaper*. Annual Report of the Chief Medical Officer on the State of Public Health. London: Department of Health.

Chief Medical Officer (2006) *On the State of Public Health*. Annual Report of the Chief Medical Officer 2005. London: Department of Health.

Citrome, L., Jaffe, A., Levine, J., Allingham, B. and Robinson, J. (2003) Antipsychotic medications treatment and new prescriptions for insulin and oral hypoglycaemics, *European Neuropsychopharmacology*, 13 (Suppl.4) S306.

Coggon, D., Rose, G. and Barker, D. (2003) *Epidemiology for the Uninitiated*, 5th edn. London: BMJ Books.

Coker, R.J., Mounier-Jack, S. and Martin, R. (2007) Public health law and tuberculosis control in Europe, *Public Health*, 121: 266–73.

Combs, D.R. and Advocat, C. (2000) Antipsychotic medication and smoking prevalence in acutely hospitalized patients with chronic schizophrenia, *Schizophrenia Research*, 46(2) 129–37.

Connolly, M. and Kelly, C. (2005) Lifestyle and physical health in schizophrenia, *Advances in Psychiatric Treatment*, 11(2) 125–32.

Craig, R. and Shelton, N. (eds) (2008) *Health Survey for England Volume 1 Healthy Lifestyles: Knowledge, Attitudes and Behaviour*. The Health and Social Care Information Centre.

Cullen, L. (2004) Nursing guidelines for ECT Appendix VII, in A. Scott (ed.) *The ECT Handbook*, 2nd edn. The Third Report of the Royal College of Psychiatrists' Special Committee on ECT Council Report CR128, January.

Currie, L., Morrell, C. and Scrivener, R. (2003) *Clinical Governance: An RCN Resource Guide*. London: Royal College of Nursing.

Daniels, L. (2002) Diet and coronary heart disease, *Nursing Standard*, 16(43) 47–54.

Daumit, G.L., Goldberg, R.W., Anthony, C., Dickerson, F., Brown, C., Kreyenbuhl, J., Wohlheiter, K. and Dixon, L. (2005) Physical activity patterns in adults with severe mental illness, *Journal of Nervous and Mental Disease*, 193(10) 641–6.

David, A. (1990) Insight and psychosis, *British Journal of Psychiatry*, 156: 798–808.

Day, J.C., Wood, G., Dewey, M. and Bentall, R.P. (1995) A self-rating scale for measuring neuroleptic side-effects. Validation in a group of schizophrenic patients, *British Journal of Psychiatry*, 166(5) 650–3.

De Freitas, B. and Schwartz, G. (1979) Effects of caffeine on chronic psychiatric patients, *American Journal of Psychiatry*, 136(10) 1337–8.

Dean, J., Todd, G., Morrow, H. and Sheldon, K. (2001) Mum, I used to be good looking . . . look at me now: the physical health needs of adults with mental health problems: The perspectives of users, carers and front-line staff, *International Journal of Mental Health Promotion*, 3(4) 16–24.

Deans, C. and Meocevic, E. (2006) Attitudes of registered psychiatric nurses towards patients diagnosed with borderline personality disorder, *Advances in Contemporary Mental Health Nursing*, 21(1) February/March.

Desai, H.D., Seabolt, J. and Jann, M.W. (2001) Smoking in patients receiving psychotropic medications: a pharmacokinetic perspective, *CNS Drugs*, 15(6) 469–94.

DH (Department of Health) (1999a) *Saving Lives: Our Healthier Nation: 4.2 Communities: Tackling the Wider Causes of Ill-health*. London: The Stationery Office.

DH (Department of Health) (1999b) *National Service Framework for Mental Health*. London: The Stationery Office.

DH (Department of Health) (2000a) *Coronary Heart Disease: National Service Framework for Coronary Heart Disease – Modern Standards and Service Models*. London: The Stationery Office.

DH (Department of Health) (2000b) *National Service Framework for Coronary Heart Disease*. London: The Stationery Office.

DH (Department of Health) (2001a) *Exercise Referral Systems: A National Quality Assurance Framework*. London: The Stationery Office.

DH (Department of Health) (2001b) *National Service Framework for Diabetes: Standards*. London: The Stationery Office.

DH (Department of Health) (2002a) *Health Improvement and Prevention. National Service Frameworks A Practical Aid to Implementation in Primary Care*. London: The Stationery Office.

DH (Department of Health) (2002b) *National Suicide Prevention Strategy for England*. London: The Stationery Office.

DH (Department of Health) (2003) *Five a Day*, http://www.dh.gov.uk/en/Publichealth/Healthimprovement/FiveADay/FiveADaygeneralinformation/index.htm

DH (Department of Health) (2004a) *At Least Five a Week: Evidence of the Impact of Physical Activity and its Relationship to Health*. A report from the Chief Medical Officer DH London http://www.dh.gov.uk/en/Publicationsandstatistics/Publications/PublicationsPolicyAndGuidance/DH_4080994

DH (Department of Health) (2004b) *Mental Health Policy Implementation Guide – Developing Positive Practice to*

Support the Safe and Therapeutic Management of Aggression and Violence in Mental Health In-patient Settings. Crown Copyright

DH (Department of Health) (2006a) *The Chief Medical Officer on the state of public health Annual Report 2005.* Crown Copyright.

DH (Department of Health) (2006b) *Turning the Corner: Improving Diabetes Care.* Crown Copyright

DH (Department of Health) (UK) (2007) *Salt,* http://www.dh.gov.uk/en/Healthcare/NationalServiceFrameworks/Bloodpressure/DH_4084299, accessed 22 July 2009.

DH (Department of Health) (2008a) *Health Inequalities,* http://www.dh.gov.uk/en/Publichealth/Healthinequalities/index.htm

DH (Department of Health) (2008b) *No more than 6g,* http://www.salt.gov.uk/no_more_than_6.html, accessed 5 January 2009.

Diabetes UK (2006) *Care Recommendation – Self-monitoring of Blood Glucose (SMBG),* http://www.diabetes.org.uk/About_us/Our_Views/Position_statements/Self-monitoring_of_blood_glucose/, accessed 22 July 2009.

Diabetes UK (2008b) *Care Recommendations: New Diagnostic Criteria for Diabetes,* http://www.diabetes.org.uk/en/About_us/Our_Views/Care_recommendations/New_diagnostic_criteria_for_diabetes_/, accessed 5 January 2009.

Diabetes UK (2008a) *Measure Up Campaign,* http://www.diabetes.org.uk, accessed 5 January 2009.

Dixon, L, Weiden, P., Delahanty, J., Goldberg, R., Postrado, L., Lucksted, A. and Lehman, A. (2000) Prevalence and correlates of diabetes in national schizophrenia samples, *Schizophrenia Bulletin,* 26(4) 903–12.

Doll, R., Peto, R., Boreham, J. and Sutherland, I. (2005) Mortality from cancer in relation to smoking: 50 years observations on British doctors, *British Journal of Cancer,* 92: 426–9.

Dougherty, L. and Lister, S. (eds) (2008) *The Royal Marsden Hospital Manual of Clinical Nursing Procedures Student Edition.* Oxford: Wiley Blackwell.

Dratcu, L., Grandison, A., McKay, G. *et al.* (2007) Clozapine-resistant psychosis, smoking, and caffeine: managing the neglected effects of substances that our patients consume every day, *American Journal of Therapeutic,* 14(3) 314–18.

DRC (Disability Rights Commission) (2003) *Coming Together – Mental Health Service Users and Disability Rights.* Stratford-upon-Avon: DRC.

DRC (Disability Rights Commission) (2006) Part I of the DRC's Formal Investigation Report *Equal Treatment: Closing the Gap. A formal investigation into physical health inequalities experienced by people with learning disabilities and/or mental health problems* : 34. Stratford-upon-Avon: DRC.

Estes, M. (2002) *Health Assessment and Physical Examination,* 2nd edn. Albany, NY: Delmar/Thomson Learning.

European Commission (2002) *Public Health,* http://ec.europa.eu/health/ph_determinants/life_style/Tobacco/tobacco_en.htm, accessed 4 December 2008.

European Society of Hypertension (2003) European Society of Hypertension – European Society of Cardiology Guidelines for the management of Arterial Hypertension, *Guidelines Committee Journal of Hypertension,* 21: 1011–53.

Evered, A. (2007) Understanding cholesterol and its role in heart disease, *Nursing Times,* 103(2) 28–9.

Ewles, L. (2005) *Key Topics in Public Health: Essential Briefings on Prevention and Health Promotion.* Edinburgh: Elsevier Churchill Livingstone.

Expert Consensus Group (2005) Metabolic and lifestyle issues and severe mental illness – new connections to well-being, *Journal of Psychopharmacology,* 19(6) Supplement: 118–22.

Expert Consensus Group (2003) 'Schizophrenia and Diabetes 2003' Expert Consensus Meeting, Dublin, 3–4 October 2003: consensus summary, *British Journal of Psychiatry,* 184: s112–S114.

Expert Group on Vitamins and Minerals (2003) *Safe Upper Levels for Vitamins and Minerals,* http://cot.food.gov.uk/pdfs/vitmin2003.pdf, accessed 22 December 2008.

Farnam, C.R., Zipple, A.M., Tyrrell, W., and Chittinanda P (1999) Health status risk factors of people with severe and persistent mental illness, *Journal of Psychosocial Nursing and Mental Health Services,* 37: 16–21.

Ferns, T. and Chojnacka, I. (2006) Conducting respiratory assessments in acute care, *Nursing Times,* 102(7) 53–5.

Ferrier, I.N. (1985) Water intoxication in patients with psychiatric illness, *British Medical Journal,* 291: 1594–6.

Finch, S. (2005) *Nurse Guidance for ECT*, http://www.rcn.org.uk/__data/assets/word_doc/0003/3774/1054_NURSE_GUIDANCE_ECT.doc, accessed 22 July 2009.

Focus on Mental Health (2001) *An Uphill Struggle: Poverty and Mental Health. Final Report of the Focus on Mental Health Work Programme 2000/2001*. London: Mental Health Foundation.

Food and Drug Administration Agency (FDA USA) (1997) Summary of safety-related drug labelling changes approved by FDA, http://www.fda.gov/Medwatch/safety/1997/jun97.htm

Food Standards Agency (no date) http://www.eatwell.gov.uk/healthydiet/nutritionessentials/vitaminsand-minerals/vitamine/, accessed 22 July 2009.

Garden, G. (2005) Physical examination in psychiatric practice, *Advances in Psychiatric Treatment*, 11: 142–9.

Gelder M, Gath D, Mayor, R and Cowen P (1996) Oxford Textbook of Psychiatry, 3rd Edition. Oxford University Press, p23

Giraud, V. and Roche, N. (2002) Misuse of corticosteroid metered-dose inhaler is associated with decreased asthma stability, *European Respiratory Journal*, 19: 246–51.

Glassman, A.H. and Bigger, J.T. (2001) Antipsychotic drugs: prolonged QTc Interval, Torsade de Pointes, and sudden death, *American Journal of Psychiatry*, 158: 1774–82.

Goddard, E. (2006) *General Household Survey, 2006 Smoking and Drinking Among Adults*. Cardiff: Office for National Statistics.

Gough, S. (2005) Diabetes and schizophrenia, *Practice Diabetes International*, 22: 23–6.

Gross, R. (2005) Chapter 4, *The Nervous System in Psychology: The Science of Mind and Behaviour*, 5th edn. London: Hodder Arnold.

Gubbay, J. (1992) *Smoking and the Workplace*. Norwich; The Centre for Health Policy Research, University of East Anglia.

Guy, W. (1976) *ECDEU Assessment Manual for Psychopharmacology*. Washington DC: US Department of Health, Education and Welfare.

Haddad, P. (1994) Letters – Neuroleptic malignant syndrome: may be caused by other drugs, *British Medical Journal*, 308: 200.

Hairon, N. (2007) Managing the increasing incidence of tuberculosis, *Nursing Times*, 103(14): 23–4.

Hall, J. (2007) Mental health staff attitudes towards exercise programmes, *Nursing Times*, 103(30): 30–1.

Hand, H. (2001) Myocardial infarction: part 1, *Nursing Standard*, 15(36): 45–55.

Harris, E. and Barraclough, B. (1998) Excess mortality of mental disorder, *British Journal of Psychiatry*, 173: 11–53.

Hastings, M. (ed.) (2009) *Clinical Skills Made Incredibly Easy*. London: Wolters Kluwer/Lippincott Williams and Wilkins.

Health Development Agency (2004) *Smoking and Patients with Mental Health Problems*. Health Development Agency.

Health Protection Agency (2008) *Tuberculosis in the UK: Annual report on tuberculosis surveillance in the UK*.

Healy, D. (2005) *Psychiatric Drugs Explained*, 4th edn. Edinburgh: Elsevier Churchill Livingstone.

Heine, R.J., Diamant, M., Mbanya, J.C. and Nathan, D.M. (2006) Clinical review management of hyperglycaemia in type 2 diabetes: the end of recurrent failure? *British Medical Journal*, 333: 1200–4.

Heiskanen *et al.* (2003) Metabolic syndrome in patients with schizophrenia, *Journal of Clinical Psychiatry*, 63: 575–79.

Herzlich, C. (1973) *Health and Illness*. London: Academic Press.

Himelhoch, S., Lehman, A., Kreyenbuhl, J. *et al.* (2004) Prevalence of chronic obstructive pulmonary disease among those with serious mental illness, *American Journal of Psychiatry*, 161: 2317–19.

HM Revenue and Customs (no date) BN 56 – *Tobacco Products: Changes in Duty Rates*, http://www.hmrc.gov.uk/budget2006/bn56.htm, accessed 22 July 2009.

Hoare, Z. and Lim, W.S. (2006) BMJ Learning Practice Pneumonia: update on diagnosis and management, *British Medical Journal*, 332: 1077–9.

Holmes, S. (2004) Malnutrition in hospital: an indictment of the quality of care? *British Journal of Healthcare Management*, 10(3): 82–5.

Holt, R.I. (2005) Obesity – an epidemic of the twenty-first century: an update for psychiatrists, *Journal of Psychopharmacology*, 19(supplement 6): 6–15.

Hooper, J. and Longworth, P. (2002) *Health Needs Assessment Workbook*. London: NHS Health Development Agency

Huether, S.E. and McCance, K.L. (eds) (2004) *Understanding Pathophysiology*, 3rd edn. Mosby.

Huffman, J.C., Blais, M.A. and Pirl, W.F. (2004) A comparison of clinician and patient concerns about antipsychotic side effects: a pilot study. *Journal of Nervous and Mental Disease*, 192(4): 328–30.

Hughes, J., Hatsukami, D., Mitchell, J. and Dahlgren, L. (1986) Prevalence of smoking among psychiatric outpatients, *American Journal of Psychiatry*, 143: 993–7.

Hunt, P. (2008) Diagnosing and managing patients with lung cancer, *Nursing Standard*, 22(33): 50–6.

Ingham, M. and O'Reilly, J. (2005) Assessment of nutritional status, in A. Crouch and C. Meurier (eds) *Health Assessment: Vital Notes for Nurses*. Oxford: Blackwell.

Information Centre (2006) *Statistics on Obesity, Physical Activity and Diet: England*. The Information Centre, Lifestyles Statistics.

Isbister, G.K., Buckley, N.A. and Whyte, I.M. (2007) Clinical update Serotonin toxicity: a practical approach to diagnosis and treatment, *Medical Journal of Australia*, 187(6).

Janssen Pharmaceuticals (2008) *Important Safety Information for Risperdal*, http://www.risperdal.com/risperdal/, accessed 25 November 2008.

Jeffery, A. (2003) Insulin resistance, *Nursing Standard*, 17(32): 47–53.

Jevon, P. and Ewens, B. (2001) Assessment of a breathless patient, *Nursing Standard*, 15(16): 48–53.

Jevon, P. (2007a) Blood pressure measurement. Part 3 Lying and standing blood pressure, *Nursing* Times, 103(20): 24–5.

Jevon, P. (2007b) Cardiac Monitoring Part 1: Electrocardiography (ECG), *Nursing Times*, 103(20): 26–7.

Jevon, P. (2007c) Respiratory Procedures Part 2: Measuring Peak Expiratory Flow, *Nursing Times*, 103(33): 26–7.

Jones, A. and Jones, M. (2008) Managing patients with antipsychotic drug-induced hyperprolactinaemia, *Nursing Standard*, 23(60): 48–55.

Jordan, S., Knight, J. and Pointon, D. (2004) Monitoring adverse drug reactions: scales, profiles, and checklists, *International Nursing Review*, 51(40): 208–21.

Kaplan, H.I., Sadock, B.J. and Grebb, J.A. (1994) *Kaplan and Sadock's Synopsis of Psychiatry: Behavioral Sciences, Clinical Psychiatry*, 7th edn. Baltimore, MD: Williams and Wilkins.

Kendrick, T. (1996) Cardiovascular and respiratory risk factors and symptoms among general practice patients with long-term mental illness, *British Journal of Psychiatry*, 169: 733–9.

Keogh, B. and Doyle, L. (2008) Psychopharmacological adverse effects, *Mental Health Practice*, 11(6): 2–30.

Killian, J.G., Kerr, K., Lawrence, C., Celermajer, D.S. (1999) Myocarditis and cardiomyopathy associated with clozapine, *Lancet*, 354: 1841–5.

Kindleysides, D. (2007) First aid: basic procedures for nurses, *Nursing Standard*, 21(19): 48–57.

Kohen, D. (2004) Diabetes mellitus and schizophrenia: historical perspective, *British Journal of Psychiatry*, 184(Supplement 47): s64–s66.

Kohen, D. and Bristow, M. (1996) Neuroleptic malignant syndrome, *Advances in Psychiatric Treatment*, 2: 151–7.

Koranyi, E.K. (1979) Morbidity and rate of undiagnosed physical illnesses in a psychiatric clinic population, *Archives of General Psychiatry*, 36: 414–19.

Kozier, B., Erb, G., Berman, A., Snyder, S., Lake, R. and Harvey, S. (2008a) Oxygenation, in *Fundamentals of Nursing: Concepts, Process, and Practice*, 8th edn. Upper Saddle River, NJ: Pearson Education.

Kozier, B., Erb, G., Berman, A., Snyder, S., Lake, R. and Harvey, S. (2008b) Pre-and post operative care, in *Fundamentals of Nursing: Concepts, Process, and Practice*, 8th edn. Upper Saddle River, NJ: Pearson Education.

Kozier, B., Erb, G., Berman, A., Snyder, S., Lake, R. and Harvey, S. (2008c) Vital signs, in *Fundamentals of Nursing: Concepts, Process, and Practice*, 8th edn. Upper Saddle River, NJ: Pearson Education.

Kurzthaler, I. and Fleischhacker, W. (2001) The clinical implications of weight gain in schizophrenia, *Journal of Clinical Psychiatry*, 62(suppl. 7): 32–7.

Lane, J.D. (1983) Caffeine and cardiovascular responses to stress, *Psychosomatic Medicine*, 45(5): 447–51.

Lawrence, D., Holman, J. and Jablensky, A. (2001) *Preventable Physical Illness in People with Mental Illness*. Perth: The University of Western Australia.

Le Pechoux, C., Dhermain, F., Bretel, J.J. *et al.* (2004) Modalities of radiotherapy in small cell lung cancer: thoracic radiotherapy and prophylactic cerebral irradiation, *Revue de Pneumologie Clinique*, 3S: 91–103.

Lean, M. and Wiseman, M. (2008) Editorial malnutrition in hospitals, *British Medical Journal*, 336: 290.

Levin, E. and Rezvani, A. (2000) Development of nicotinic drug therapy for cognitive disorders, *European Journal of Pharmacology*, 393(1–3): 141–6.

Lewis, G. and Appleby, L. (1988) Personality disorder: the patients psychiatrists dislike. *British Journal of Psychiatry*, 153: 44–9.

Linden, M. and Godemann, F. (2005) The differentiation between 'Lack of Insight' and 'Dysfunctional Health Beliefs' in schizophrenia, *Psychopathology*, 40(4): 236–41.

Llorente, M.D. and Urrutia, V. (2006) Diabetes, psychiatric disorders, and the metabolic effects of anti-psychotic medications, *Clinical Diabetes*, 24(1): 18–24.

Lloyd, P. and Moodley, P. (1992) Psychotropic medication and ethnicity: an inpatient survey, *Social Psychiatry and Psychiatric Epidemiology*, 27(2): 95–101.

Lobstein, T., Rigby, N. and Leach, R. (2005) Obesity in Europe – 3 International Obesity TaskForce March 2005, http://ec.europa.eu/health/ph_determinants/life_style/nutrition/documents/iotf_en.pdf, accessed 20 December 2008.

Loos, R.J. and Bouchard, C. (2003) Obesity – is it a genetic disorder? *Journal of Internal Medicine*, 254(5): 401–25.

Louch, P. (2005) Depression management in primary care, *Primary Health Care*, 15(10): 20–2.

Lowe, T. and Lubos, E. (2008) Effectiveness of weight management interventions for people with serious mental illness who receive treatment with atypical antipsychotic medications. A literature review, *Journal of Psychiatric and Mental Health Nursing*, 15(10): 857–63.

Lynn, P. (ed.) (2004) Vital signs, in *Taylor's Clinical Nursing Skills: A Nursing Process Approach*, 2nd edn. Philadelphia, PA: Lippincott Williams and Wilkins.

McCreadie, R.G. and Kelly, C. (2000) Patients with schizophrenia who smoke: private disaster, public resource, *British Journal of Psychiatry*, Editorial 176: 109.

McCreadie, R., Macdonald, E., Blacklock, C., *et al.* (1998) Dietary intake of schizophrenic patients in Nithsdale, Scotland: case-control study, *British Medical Journal*, 317: 784–5.

McFerran, T. (2008) *Oxford Dictionary of Nursing*, 5th Edn. Oxford: Oxford University Press.

McIntyre, J.S. and Romano, J. (1977) Is there a stethoscope in the house (and is it used)? *Archives of General Psychiatry*, 34: 1147–51.

McNeil, A. (2004) *Smoking and Patients with Mental Health Problems*. London: Health Development Agency.

McNeill, A. (2001) *Smoking and Mental Health – A Review of the Literature*. SmokeFree London Programme December 2001.

McQuistion, H.L., Colson, P., Yankowitz, R. and Susser, E. (1997) Tuberculosis infection among people with severe mental illness, *Psychiatric Services*, 48: 833–5.

Mackay, F., Dunn, N. and Mann, D. (1999) Antidepressants and the serotonin syndrome in general practice, *British Journal of General Practice*, 49(448): 871–4.

Mains, J., Coxall, E. and Lloyd, H. (2008) Measuring temperature, *Nursing Standard*, 22(39): 44–7.

Malarkey, L.M, and McMorrow, M.E, (2005) *Saunders Nursing Guide to Laboratory and Diagnostic Tests*. Philadelphia, PA: Elsevier Saunders.

Mallett, J. and Dougherty, L. (eds) (2000) *Manual of Clinical Nursing Procedures*, 5th edn. London: Blackwell Science.

Marder, S., Essock, S., Miller, A. *et al.* (2004) Physical health monitoring of patients with schizophrenia, *American Journal of Psychiatry*, 161(8): 1334–49.

Marks, V. (2003) The metabolic syndrome, *Nursing Standard*, 17(49): 37–44.

Mathias, C.J. and Kimber, J.R. (1999) Postural hypotension: causes, clinical features, investigation, and management, *Annual Revue of Medicine*, 50: 317–36.

Meddings, S. and Perkins, R. (2002) What 'getting better' means to staff and users of a rehabilitation service: an exploratory study, *Journal of Mental Health*, 11(3): 319–25.

Meiklejohn, C., Sanders, K. and Butler, S. (2003) Physical health care in medium secure services, *Nursing Standard*, 17(17): 33–7.

Meltzer, H., Singleton, N., Lee, A., *et al.* (2002) *The Social and Economic Circumstances of Adults with Mental Disorders*. London: The Stationery Office.

Mental Health Act Commission (1999) *Eighth Biennial Report*. London: The Stationery Office.

Mental Health Foundation (2007) Smoking and mental health, http://www.mentalhealth.org.uk/information/mental-health-a-z/smoking/, accessed 9 December 2008.

Mentality and NIMHE (2004) Healthy body and mind: promoting healthy living for people who experience mental distress; a guide for people working in primary health care teams supporting people with severe and enduring mental illness

Metherall, A., Worthington, R. and Keyte, A. (2006) Research Article – Twenty four hour medical emergency response teams in a mental health in-patient facility – New approaches for safer restraint, *Journal of Psychiatric Intensive Care*, 2(1): 21–9.

Meurier, C. (2005) The human body, in A. Crouch and C. Meurier (eds) *Health Assessment: Vital Notes for Nurses*. Oxford: Blackwell Publishing.

MHRA (2009) *Paracetamol Overdose. Medicines and Healthcare Products Regulatory Agency (MHRA)* http://www.mhra.gov.uk/Howweregulate/Medicines/Licensingofmedicines/Informationforlicenceapplicants/Guidance/OverdosesectionsofSPCs/Genericoverdosesections/Paracetamol/index.htm, accessed 22 July 2009.

Mind (1996) *Not Just Sticks and Stones: A Survey of the Stigma, Taboos and Discrimination Experienced by People with Mental Health Problems*. London: Mind.

Möller, H.J. (2000) State of the art of drug treatment of schizophrenia and the future position of the novel/atypical antipsychotics, *World Journal of Biological Psychiatry*, 1: 204–14.

Moore, T. (2007) Respiratory assessment in adults, *Nursing Standard*, 21(49): 48–56.

Morice, A.H., McGarvey, L. and Pavord, I. (2006) Recommendations for the management of cough in adults, British Thoracic Society Cough Guideline Group, *Thorax*, 61(Supplement I)i1–i24.

Muir-Cochrane, E. (2006) Medical co-morbidity risk factors and barriers to care for people with schizophrenia, *Journal of Psychiatric and Mental Health Nursing*, 13: 447–52.

Murphy, M.J., Cowan, R.L. and Sederer, L.I. (2004) *Major Adverse Drug Reactions in Blueprints Psychiatry*, 3rd edn. Philadelphia, PA: Lippincott Williams and Wilkins.

Murray, R. (2005) *Schizophrenia Research Forum Interview*, http://www.schizophreniaforum.org/for/int//Murray/murray.asp, accessed 22 July 2009.

Nash, M. (2005) Physical care skills: a training needs analysis of inpatient and community mental health nurses, *Mental Health Practice*, 9(4): 24–7.

Nash, M. (2002) Voting as a means of social inclusion for people with a mental illness, *Journal of Psychiatric and Mental Health Nursing*, 9(6): 697–703.

Nash, M. (2008) Weight ÷ Height x Age: Mental Health Nurses knowledge of basic aspects of physical care. Paper presented at the RCN European Mental Health Conference, UK, 6–7 March 2008.

National Center for Health Statistics (2007) *Data Brief – Obesity Among Adults in the United States – No Statistically Significant Change Since 2003–2004*, Centers for Disease Control and Prevention National Center for Health Statistics, http://www.cdc.gov/nchs/data/databriefs/db01.pdf, accessed 22 July 2009.

National Cholesterol Education Program (NCEP) (2002) Third Report of the National Cholesterol Education Program (NCEP) Expert Panel on Detection, Evaluation, and Treatment of High Blood Cholesterol in Adults (Adult Treatment Panel III) Final Report Circulation 2002; 106: 3143

National Collaborating Centre for Acute Care (2005) *The Diagnosis and Treatment of Lung Cancer Methods, Evidence and Guidance*. London: NICE.

National Heart, Lung and Blood Institute (2007a) *National Asthma Education and Prevention Program Expert Panel Report 3: Guidelines for the Diagnosis and Management of Asthma*, Full Report. US Department of Health and Human Services.

National Heart, Lung and Blood Institute (2007b) *Expert Panel Report 3 (EPR3) Guidelines for the Diagnosis and Management of Asthma Section 3, The Four Components of Asthma Management*. Bethesda, MD: US Department of Health and Human Services National Institutes of Health.

National Institute for Health Research (2007) *Pemetrexed Disodium (Alimta) for the First Line Treatment of Advanced Non-small Cell Lung Cancer*. Birmingham: National Horizon Scanning Centre.

National Patient Safety Agency (2008) *Rapid Response Report NPSA/2008/RRR010: Resuscitation in Mental Health and Learning Disability Settings*. National Patient Safety Agency.

NCCCC (The National Collaborating Centre for Chronic Conditions) (2004) Prevalence of COPD Introduction, *Thorax*, 59 (Supplement I): 1–232.

NDARC (National Drug and Alcohol Research Centre (no date) *Fact sheet: Caffeine*. http://ndarc.med.unsw.edu.au/NDARCWeb.nsf/resources/NDARCFact_Drugs6/$file/caffeine+fact+sheet.pdf, accessed 24 October 2008.

NICE (National Institute of Health and Clinical Excellence) (2002) *Clinical Guideline 1 Schizophrenia Core Interventions in the Treatment and Management of Schizophrenia in Primary and Secondary Care*. London: National Collaborating Centre for Mental Health.

NICE (2004) *Clinical Guideline 12 Chronic Obstructive Pulmonary Disease Management of Chronic Obstructive Pulmonary Disease in Adults in Primary and Secondary Care Developed by the National Collaborating Centre for Chronic Conditions*. London: NICE.

NICE (2005) Clinical Guideline 25 Violence: The Short-term Management of Disturbed/Violent Behaviour in In-patient Psychiatric Settings and Emergency Departments. London: NICE and the National Collaborating Centre for Nursing and Supportive Care.

NICE (2006a) *Clinical Guideline 38 Bipolar Disorder: The Management of Bipolar Disorder in Adults, Children and Adolescents, in Primary and Secondary Care*. London: NICE and the National Collaborating Centre for Mental Health.

NICE (2006b) *Clinical Guideline 33 Tuberculosis: Clinical Diagnosis and Management of Tuberculosis, and Measures for its Prevention and Control*. London: NICE.

NICE (2006c) *Clinical Guideline 43 Obesity: The Prevention, Identification, Assessment and Management of Overweight and Obesity in Adults and Children*. National Institute for Health and Clinical Excellence National Collaborating Centre for Primary Care.

NICE (2007a) *Clinical Guideline 50 Acutely Ill Patients in Hospital: Recognition of and Response to Acute Illness in Adults in Hospital*. London: NICE.

NICE (2007b) *Clinical Guideline 23 Depression*. London: NICE.

NICE (2008) *Clinical Guideline 66 Type 2 Diabetes: The Management of Type 2 Diabetes* (update). London: NICE.

NICE (2009) *Schizophrenia Core Interventions in the Treatment and Management of Schizophrenia in Primary and Secondary Care* (update) National Clinical Practice Guideline Number 8. London: NICE.

Nicol, M., Bavin, C., Bedford-Turner, S., Cronin, P. and Rawlings-Anderson, K. (2003) *Essential Nursing Skills*, 2nd edn. Edinburgh: Mosby.

Nicol, M., Bavin, C., Bedford-Turner, S., Cronin, P. and Rawlings-Anderson, K. (2004) Observation and monitoring, in *Essential Nursing Skills*, 2nd edn. Edinburgh: Mosby.

NMC (Nursing and Midwifery Council) (2007) *The Code: Standards of Conduct, Performance and Ethics for Nurses and Midwives*. London: NMC.

Nocon, A. and Sayce, L. (2006) Closing the gap: tackling physical health inequalities in primary care, in C. Jackson and K. Hill (eds) *Mental Health Today: A Handbook*. Pavillion Publishing.

Novartis (2008) CLOZARIL (*clozapine*) Tablets Prescribing Information http://www.pharma.us.novartis.com/product/pi/pdf/Clozaril.pdf, accessed 31/7/09.

Obesity Focused (2008) *Setting Standards in the Definition of Obesity*, available at http://www.obesityfocused.com/articles/about-obesity/definition-of-obesity.php, accessed 31 July 2009.

O'Brien, P. and Oyebode, F. (2003) Psychotropic medication and the heart, *Advances in Psychiatric Treatment*, 9: 414–23.

ODPM (Office of the Deputy Prime Minister) (2004) *Mental Health and Social Exclusion: Social Exclusion Unit Report*. London: Social Exclusion Unit.

Oehl, M., Hummer, M. and Fleischhacker, W.W. (2000) Compliance with antipsychotic treatment, *Acta Psychiatrica Scandinavia*, 102(Suppl. 407): 83–6.

ONS (Office for National Statistics) (2004) *Life Expectancy: More Aged 70 and 80 than Ever Before*, http://www.statistics.gov.uk/cci/nugget.asp?id=881, accessed 22 July 2009.

ONS (2005) *General Household Survey*. London: Office of National Statistics.

Osborn, D.P.J., Levy, G., Nazareth, I., *et al.* (2007) Relative risk of cardiovascular and cancer mortality in people with severe mental illness from the United Kingdom's General Practice Research Database, *Archives of General Psychiatry*, 64: 242–9.

Ovbiagele, B. (2008) Microalbuminuria: risk factor and potential therapeutic target for stroke? *Journal of the Neurological Sciences*, 271(1–2): 1–8.

Oxford Dictionary of Biology, 4th edition (2000) Oxford: Oxford University Press.

Pallavi Lanjewar, P., Pathak, V. and Lokhandwala, Y. (2004) Editorial Issues in QT interval measurement, *Indian Pacing Electrophysiology Journal*, 4(4): 156–61.

Palmer, R. (2004) An overview of diabetic ketoacidosis, *Nursing Standard*, 19(1): 42–4.

Parks, J., Svendsen, D., Singer, P. and Foti, M. (2006) Foreword, in *Morbidity and Mortality of People with Serious Mental Illness*. National Association of State Mental Health Program Directors (NASMHPD) Medical Directors Council.

Patel, P. and Bristow, G. (1987) Postoperative neuroleptic malignant syndrome: a case report, *Canadian Journal of Anaesthesia*, 35(5): 515–18.

Patkar, A., Gopalakrishnan, R., Lundy, A., *et al.* (2002) Relationship between tobacco smoking and positive and negative symptoms in schizophrenia, *Journal of Nervous and Mental Disease*, 190: 604–10.

Patton, D. (2008) Treatment modalities in psychiatric nursing practice, in J. Morrisey, B. Keogh and L. Doyle (eds) *Psychiatric/Mental Health Nursing: An Irish Perspective*. Dublin: Gill and Macmillan.

Pedder, L. (1998) Training-needs analysis, *Nursing Standard*, 13(6): 50–6.

Peet, M. (2002) Essential fatty acids: theoretical aspects and treatment implications for schizophrenia and depression, *Advances in Psychiatric Treatment*, 8: 223–9.

Peet, M. and Stokes, C. (2005) Omega-3 fatty acids in the treatment of psychiatric disorders, *Drugs*, 65(8): 1051–9.

Perry, L. (2007) The use of body measurements to assess nutritional status, http://www.nursingtimes.net/nursing-practice-clinical-research/the-use-of-body-measurements-to-assess-nutritional-status/199379.article, accessed 22 July 2009.

Phelan, M., Stradins, L. and Morrison, S. (2001) Physical health of people with severe mental illness, *British Medical Journal*, 322: 443–4.

Pirl, W.F., Greer, J.A., Weissgarber, C., Liverant, G. and Safren, S.A. (2005) Screening for infectious diseases among patients in a state psychiatric hospital, *Psychiatric Services*, 56: 1614–16.

Pope, B. (2008) How to perform 3-or 5-lead monitoring, Nursing FindArticles.com, http://findarticles.com/p/articles/mi_qa3689/is_200204/ai_n9074027, accessed 18 November 2008.

Potter, P. and Perry, A. (2005) Vital signs, in *Fundamentals of Nursing*, 6th edn. St Louis, MO: Elsevier Mosby

Price, C., Seong, W. and Rutherford, I. (2000) Advanced nursing practice: an introduction to physical assessment, *British Journal of Nursing*, 9(22): 2292–6.

Prignot, J. (1987) Review Article – Quantification and chemical markers of tobacco-exposure, *European Journal of Respiratory Disease*, 70: 1–7.

Prochaska, J.O. and DiClemente, C.C. (1983) Stages and processes of self-change of smoking: toward an integrative model of change. *Journal of Consulting and Clinical Psychology*, 51(3): 390–5.

Provan, D. (ed.) (2007) *Oxford Handbook of Clinical and Laboratory Investigation*. Oxford; Oxford University Press.

Public Health Agency of Canada (2002) *A Report on Mental Illnesses in Canada*. http://www.phac-aspc.gc.ca/publicat/miic-mmac/chap_1-eng.php, accessed 22 July 2009.

Raw, M., Mc Neill, A., West, R. (1998) Smoking cessation guidelines for health professionals. A guide to effective smoking cessation interventions for the health care system, *Thorax*, 53(Supplement 5): S1–S18.

Raw, M., McNeill, A., West, R., Armstrong, A. and Arnott, D. (2005) *Nicotine Assisted Reduction to Stop (NARS). Guidance for Health Professionals on this New Indication for Nicotine Replacement Therapy*. London: ASH.

Rayner, C. and Prigmore, S. (2008) Illicit drug use and its effects on the lungs, *Nursing Times*, 104(9): 40–4.

Reilly, J.G., Ayis, A., Ferrier, I.N., Jones, S.J. and Thomas, S.H.L. (2002) Thioridazine and sudden unexplained death in psychiatric in-patients, *British Journal of Psychiatry*, 180: 515–22.

Resuscitation Council UK (2005) *Adult Basic Life Support Algorithm*, http://www.resus.org.uk/pages/inhresus.pdf, accessed 22 July 2009.

Resuscitation Council UK (2004) *Intermediate Life Support Course Manual*. London: RCUK.

Rettenbacher, M., Ebenbichler, C., Hofer, A., *et al.* (2006) Early changes of plasma lipids during treatment with atypical antipsychotics. Short Report, *International Clinical Psychopharmacology*, 21(6): 369–72.

Roberts, L., Roalfe, A., Wilson, S. and Lester, H. (2007) Physical health care of patients with schizophrenia in primary care: a comparative study, *Family Practice*, 24: 34–40.

Robson, D. and Gray, R. (2007) Physical health problems in people with serious mental illness, *International Journal of Nursing Studies*, 44(3): 457–66.

Roper, N., Logan, W.W., Tierney, A.J. (1996) *The Elements of Nursing*, 3rd edn. Edinburgh: Churchill Livingstone.

Royal College of Psychiatrists (2007) Schizophrenia. Changing Minds, http://www.rcpsych.ac.uk/default.aspx?page=1643, accessed 17 March 2009.

Rushforth, H., Warner, J., Burge, D. and Glasper, E. (1998) Nursing physical assessment: implications for practice, *British Journal of Nursing*, 7(16): 965–70.

Ruxton, C. (2004) Health benefits of omega-3 fatty acids, *Nursing Standard*, 18(48): 38–42.

Samar, A. (1999) The pathogenesis of atherosclerosis, in N. Jairath (ed.) *Coronary Heart Disease and Risk Factor Management: A Nursing Perspective*. Philadelphia, PA: WB Saunders.

Samaraseka, U. (2007) Staffing issues affecting care on acute psychiatric wards, Special Report, *The Lancet*, 370(9582): 119–20.

Saracci, R. (1997) The world health organisation needs to reconsider its definition of health, *British Medical Journal*, 314: 1409.

Sayce, L. (2000) *From Psychiatric Patient to Citizen: Overcoming Discrimination and Social Exclusion*. London: Macmillan.

Sayce, L. (2001) Editorial: *Social inclusion and mental health*. Psychiatric Bulletin, 25: 121–23.

Select Committee on Public Accounts (2002) *Ninth Report Tackling Obesity in England* (HC 421). London: Parliamentary Copyright.

Silva, E. (1999) Rapid tranquillisation in isolated units, i.m. medication preferable to i.v, *Journal of Psychopharmacology*, 13: 200–1.

Silverstone, T., Smith, G. and Goodall, E. (1988) Prevalence of obesity in patients receiving depot antipsychotics, *British Journal of Psychiatry*, 153: 214–17.

Singleton, N., Bumpstead, R., O'Brien, M. *et al.* (2000) *Psychiatric Morbidity among Adults Living in Private Households Prevalence of Longstanding Physical Complaints by Probable Psychotic Disorder*. The report of a survey carried out by Social Survey Division of the Office for National Statistics on behalf of the Department of Health, the Scottish Executive and the National Assembly for Wales. London: The Stationery Office.

Smith, S.F., Duell, D.J., Martin, B.C. (2008a) Intravenous therapy, in *Clinical Nursing Skills Basic to Advanced Skills*, 7th edn. London: Pearson Education.

Smith, M., Hopkins, D., Peveler, R.C., Holt, *et al.* (2008b) First- v. second-generation antipsychotics and risk for diabetes in schizophrenia: systematic review and meta-analysis, *British Journal of Psychiatry*, 192: 406–11.

Social Exclusion Unit (2004) *The Role of Health and Social Care Professionals in Promoting Social Inclusion Factsheet 2*. London: Office of the Deputy Prime Minister. Crown Copyright 2004.

Swan, P. and Raphael, B. (1995) *Ways Forward: National Aboriginal and Torres Strait Islander Mental Health Policy National Consultancy Report Part 1*, http://www.aodgp.gov.au/internet/main/publishing.nsf/Content/mental-pubs-w-wayforw-toc~mental-pubs-w-wayforw-exe, accessed 22 July 2009.

Taylor, D., Paton, C. and Kerwin, R. (2005) *The Maudsley Prescribing Guidelines 2005–2006*. London: Taylor and Francis.

Theisen, F.M., Cichon, S., Linden, A., *et al.* (2001) Clozapine and weight gain, *American Journal of Psychiatry*, 158: 816.

Timmer, R.T. and Sands, J.F. (1999) Lithium intoxication, *Journal of the American Society of Nephrology*, 110: 666–74.

TNS (2007) *Attitudes to Mental Illness*, 2007 Report. TNS, Crown Copyright.

Tonkin, R. (2003) *The X Factor: Obesity and the Metabolic Syndrome*. London: The Science and Public Affairs Forum.

Took, M. (2001) *Physical care needs of people with a severe mental illness*. National Schizophrenia Fellowship Policy Statement, London.

Tortora, G. and Derrickson, B. (2006) *Principles of Anatomy and Physiology*, 11th edn. New York/Chichester: Wiley International.

Tough, J. (2004) Assessment and treatment of chest pain, *Nursing Standard*, 18(37): 45–53.

Trim, J. (2004) Performing a comprehensive physiological assessment, *Nursing Times*, 100(50): 38–42.

Tschoner, A., Engl, J., Laimer, M. *et al.* (2007) Metabolic side effects of antipsychotic medication review article, *International Journal of Clinical Practice*, 61(8): 1356–70.

Twinn, S., Roberts, B. and Andrews, S. (1996) *Community Health Care Nursing: Principles for Practice*. Oxford: Butterworth-Heinemann.

UK Lung Cancer coalition (2005) Factsheet, available at http://www.uklcc.org.uk/word/uklccresearch-factsheet.doc, accessed 28 November 200.

Varchol, D.A. and Raynor, J. (2008) Biological basis for understanding psychopharmacology, in *Essentials of Psychiatric Mental Health Nursing: A Communication Approach to Evidence-Based Care*. Elsevier Health Sciences.

Waddington, J.L., Youssef, H.A. and Kinsella, A. (1998) Mortality in schizophrenia. Antipsychotic poly-pharmacy and absence of adjunctive anticholinergics over the course of a 10-year prospective study, *British Journal of Psychiatry*, 173: 325–9.

Walsh, D. and Daly, A. (2004) *Mental Illness in Ireland 1750–2002. Reflections on the Rise and Fall of Institutional Care Health*. Dublin: Research Board.

Wanless, D. (2004) *Securing Good Health for the Whole Population: Final Report*. London: HMSO.

Ward, G. (1997) *Making Headlines, Mental Health and the National Press*. London: Health Education Authority.

Watkins, P. (2003) ABC of diabetes. Cardiovascular disease, hypertension and lipids, *British Medical Journal*. 326, 19 April.

Watson, D. (2008a) Pneumonia 1: recognising signs and symptoms, *Nursing Times*, 104(4): 28–9.

Watson, D. (2008b) Pneumonia 2: effective assessment and management, *Nursing Times*, 104(5): 30–1.

Waugh, A. and Grant, A. (2006) *Ross and Wilson Anatomy and Physiology in Health and* Illness, 10th edn. Philadelphia, PA: Churchill Livingstone.

Webster, R. and Thompson, D. (2006) Disorders of the cardio-vascular system, in M. Alexander, J. Fawcett and P. Runciman P (eds) *Nursing Practice Hospital and Home. The Adult*, 3rd edn. Philadehia, PA: Churchill Livinstone.

Weiden, P., Mackell, J. and McDonnell, D. (2004) Obesity as a risk factor for antipsychotic non-compliance, *Schizophrenia Research*, 66(1): 51–7.

West, R. (2004) ABC of smoking cessation. Assessment of dependence and motivation to stop smoking, *British Medical Journal*, 328: 338–9.

WHO (World Health Organization) (1948) *Constitution of the World Health Organization*, http://www.searo.who.int/LinkFiles/About_SEARO_const.pdf, accessed 22 July 2009.

WHO (1998) *Health Promotion Glossary*. Geneva; World Health Organization.

WHO (1999) Definition, diagnosis and classification of diabetes mellitus and its complications: report of a WHO Consultation. Part 1: diagnosis and classification of diabetes mellitus. Geneva: World Health Organization.

WHO (2000a) *Diabetes Prevalence World Wide*, http://www.who.int/diabetes/facts/world_figures/en/, accessed 3 July 2007.

WHO (2000b) Obesity: preventing and managing the global epidemic Part 1 the problem of overweight and obesity WHO Technical Report Series, No. 894, http://whqlibdoc.who.int/trs/WHO_TRS_894_ (part1).pdf, accessed 19 December 2008.

WHO (2001) *Conquering Depression: You Can Get Out of the Blues*, http://www.searo.who.int/en/section1174/ section1199/section1567_6741.htm, accessed 22 July 2009.

WHO (2003) *Investing in Mental Health*, http://www.who.int/mental_health/media/investing_mnh_ final.pdf, accessed 22 July 2009.

WHO (2004a) *Promoting Mental Health; Concepts, Emerging Evidence, Practice. Summary Report*. A Report of the World Health Organization, Department of Mental Health and Substance Abuse in collaboration with the Victorian Health Promotion Foundation and the University of Melbourne. Geneva: WHO.

WHO (2004b) *The tobacco atlas, Part 6 table A: The demographics of tobacco*, http://www.who.int/tobacco/ en/atlas40.pdf, accessed 22 July 2009.

WHO (2006) *BMI Classification*, http://www.who.int/bmi/index.jsp?introPage=intro_3.html, accessed 5 January 2009.

WHO (2008a) *Mental Health: The Bare Facts*. http://www.who.int/mental_health/en/, accessed 22 July 2009.

WHO (2008b) *Nutrition for Health and Development*, http://www.who.int/nutrition/en/, accessed 22 December 2008.

WHO (2008c) *Reduction of Micronutrient Malnutrition Micronutrients*, http://www.who.int/nutrition/topics/ micronutrients/en/index.html, accessed 22 December 2008.

WHO (2008d) Tobacco Free Initiative. Why is tobacco a public health priority? http://www.who.int/ tobacco/health_priority/en/index.html, accessed 22 July 2009.

WHO/FAO (2003) WHO technical report series; 916 Diet, nutrition and the prevention of chronic diseases: report of a joint WHO/FAO expert consultation, Geneva, 28 January–1 February 2002.

Williams, B., Poulter, N.R., Brown, M.J., *et al.* (2004) British Hypertension Society Guidelines: Guidelines for management of hypertension: report of the fourth working party of the British Hypertension Society, 2004 – BHS IV, *Journal of Human Hypertension*, 18: 139–85.

Williams, K. and Pinfold, V. (2006) *Side Effects: Mental Health Service Users' Experiences of the Side Effects of Antipsychotic Medication*. Kingston upon Thames: Rethink.

Yamey, G. (1999) The press reviews struck off, but why? *British Medical Journal*, 319: 791.

Yusuf, S., Hawken, S., Ounpuu, S., *et al.*, (2005) Obesity and the risk of myocardial infraction in 27 000 participants from 52 countries: a case-control study, *The Lancet*, 366: 1640–9.

Index

Related books from Open University Press

Purchase from www.openup.co.uk or order through your local bookseller

NURSING IN CHILD AND ADOLESCENT MENTAL HEALTH

Nisha Dogra and Sharon Leighton

This book focuses on child and adolescent mental health (CAMH) for nurses training and working in this field. The authors explore the various roles CAMH nurses fulfil and consider how these roles might be undertaken with confidence.

Drawing upon both the academic evidence available, and grounded in the reality of clinical practice, the book looks at how to assess the different issues and the various interventions used in practice. The authors consider the effect of child and family development on mental health, as well as broader factors influencing mental health and well-being. Among the core issues considered are:

- Definitions and consequences of mental health, illness and stigma
- Child development
- Legislative frameworks
- Assessment skills
- Therapeutic work: individual counselling, cognitive behavioural therapy, family work and medication
- Clinical governance and supervision
- Research

Nursing in Child and Adolescent Mental Health is relevant to nurses at all levels, but is especially useful to postgraduate nurses and nurses in specialist child and adolescent mental health services (SCAMHS). Other professional staff will also find it useful.

Contents

Introduction – Defining mental health and mental illness – Child and family development – The aetiology of child mental health problems – Legal and ethical considerations in CAMH – Nursing assessment in CAMHS – Counselling and the therapeutic use of self – Family work and CAMHS nursing – Cognitive behavioural therapy and the CAMH nurse – Nurse prescribing and medication management in CAMHS – Inpatient CAMH nursing: two different models of care – Multi-agency working – Working with vulnerable children and young people – Clinical governance, audit and supervision – Nurses and CAMH research – Developing mental health services for children and adolescents – Index

2009 264pp
978–0–335–23463–9 (Paperback) 978–0–335–23462–2 (Hardback)

AN INTRODUCTION TO MENTAL HEALTH NURSING

Nick Wrycraft

Full of insights into what it's like to be a mental health nursing student, including direct quotes from current students!

This engaging new textbook provides a student focused introduction to the main issues and themes in mental health nursing. The book requires no previous knowledge and the content has been carefully chosen to reflect the most significant aspects of this important and rewarding area of nursing.

The book includes specific chapters on:

- Social inclusion and the Ten Essential Shared Capabilities
- Mental health promotion
- Mental health at different stages of the life course
- Physical health issues in mental health settings
- Mental health law
- Therapeutic interventions, specifically Cognitive Behavioural Therapy (CBT) and psychoanalytic/ psychodynamic approaches
- The concept of recovery

Scenarios and exercises are used to demonstrate integration of theory and practice. These can be easily linked to your placement experience and overall learning and development. Readers are encouraged to develop an analytical and investigative approach to their studies.

Other important areas covered in the book include the National Service Framework (NSF) for Mental Health, the Care Programme Approach (CPA) and the Tidal Model of mental health nursing.

Introduction to Mental Health Nursing is the perfect introduction for all nursing students with an interest in a career in mental health nursing.

Contributors
Geoffrey Amoateng, Amanda Blackhall, Alyson Buck, David A. Hingley, David Dean Holyoake, Richard Khoo, Mark McGrath, Mary Northrop, Tim Schafer, Julie Teatheredge, James Trueman, Henck Van- Bilsen, Steve Wood.

Contents
Background to mental health nurse training – Learning on practice placements – Mental health and recognition of mental illness – Risk assessment: Practicing accountably and responsibly – Mental Health Nursing and the Law – Mental health promotion – Section 2 – Children and adolescent mental health – Adult mental health services in the community – Secure inpatient and forensic mental health care for adults – The mental health of older adults – Section 3 – Physical health issues in mental health practice – CBTN – Psychodynamic and psychoanalytic therapeutic interventions in mental health – Recovery – Social inclusion – Conclusion

2009 368pp
ISBN-13: 978–0–335–23358–8   (ISBN-10: 033–5–23358–9) Paperback
ISBN-13: 978–0–335–23357–1   (ISBN-10: 033–5–23357–0) Hardback

THE ART AND SCIENCE OF MENTAL HEALTH NURSING
SECOND EDITION

Ian Norman and Iain Ryrie

This second edition has been extensively revised to incorporate changes to the UK policy context of mental health nursing, the legal framework of mental health care and the 2006 Chief Nursing Officer's Review of Mental Health Nursing, From Values to Action. Throughout the text, readers are encouraged to draw upon the evidence base to inform the delivery of high quality mental health care.

Key features:

- Written by an expert group of clinicians and researchers drawn from a range of disciplines
- Provides readers with an authoritative account of mental health care policies and practice
- Integrates service-users' views and highlights the role of nurses in helping them find meaning and purpose
- Emphasises the importance of understanding lifestyle interventions to promote mental health and the public health role of the mental health nurse
- Case studies are integrated throughout the text to illustrate the practical application of the material
- Superb pedagogy aids learning though overviews, conclusions, questions for reflection and discussion, as well as an annotated bibliography guiding the reader towards more detailed reading

Contents

Mental health – Mental disorder – Future directions in mental health promotion and public mental health – Mental health nursing: origins and traditions – Recovery and social inclusion – The policy and service context of mental health nursing – Law and ethics of mental health nursing – Functional teams and whole systems – Service improvement – Assessment – Assessing and managing risk – Modern milieus: psychiatric inpatient treatment in the 21st century – Strategies for living and lifestyle options – Psychosocial interventions – Physical health care and serious mental illness – Psychopharmacology – Complementary and alternative therapies – The person with a perceptual disorder – The person with an affective/mood disorder – The person with an anxiety disorder – The person with an eating disorder – The person with co-existing mental health and substance misuse problems ('dual diagnosis') – Mental health problems in childhood and adolescence – The person with dementia – Forensic mental health care – The person with a personality disorder – Engaging clients in their care and treatment – Problems, goals and care planning – Self-help – Behavioural techniques – Cognitive techniques – Medication management to concordance – Therapeutic management of aggression and violence – Nursing people who self-harm or are suicidal – Future directions: taking recovery into society

2009   744pp
978–0–335–22293–3 (Paperback)

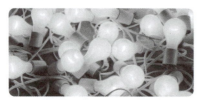
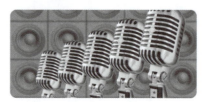
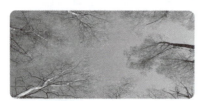
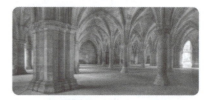
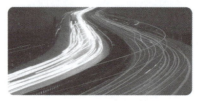
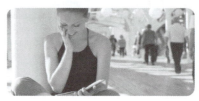
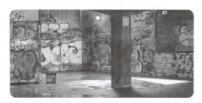